# Intermittent Fast Meal Planning

## GINNY McKEIN

A well organized weekly plan easy even for beginners.

Delicious Recipes with photos.

You will have a Intermittent Fasting 16/8

for woman over 50

# Table of content

# Introduction

Are you looking for a healthy diet?
Are you looking for an easy diet to put into practice?
You don't want to give up your traditional food
Do you want to improve your health?
Do you want to live longer?
Do you want to stay young and strong?

This is not really a diet, but a food program that gives you maximum freedom: you can continue to eat what you like, abstaining completely or partially only a few hours a day or just a few days a week or a month.

Everyone can choose between the various variants the one: that is easier for himself and his lifestyle.

You can choose between these variants: 16/8-5/2-E.S.E.-5/30
and you will have the following advantages:

- Activates stem cell-based renewal in the body for anti-aging benefits
- Lose weight and reduce abdominal fat for better health
- Extend your healthy life with simple daily changes
- Prevents bone and muscle loss
- Build your resistance to diabetes, cardiovascular disease, Alzheimer's disease and cancer.

# Chapter 1$^{st}$

## A step ahead intermittent fast diet, to loss weight for a healthy lifestyle

Intermittent fasting should not be confused with extreme and reckless forms of fasting recommended by fanatics of "detoxifying" diets or by self-proclaimed new age gurus who are fan of hydrocolontherapy. When we talk about intermittent fasting we intend to indicate a series of protocols based on short-term fasts, with the aim of improving the health of the subject.
As we will explain, it has nothing to do with the ascetic fasting of ten days based on water and lemon, those able to produce important problems, first of all a loss of precious lean mass once the 72 hours of abstinence from the food.
Those who like to interpret human behavior in the light of evolution maintain that spending prolonged periods without food intake, alternated with windows in which food is freely consumed, can accurately mimic the conditions in which our species has evolved and therefore it can best support the physiological mechanisms developed during the evolutionary pathway. On the other hand, up to two or three generations ago the food available was not so abundant and often individuals, by force, spent relatively long periods without eating.
The recent availability of low-priced food, high caloric content and mediocre nutritional properties has created a condition whereby our body is ill-adapted, a situation underlying the epidemic of obesity and diabetes that is spreading in the industrialized world. Suggestive hypotheses that require further study, without the enthusiastic simplifications that some followers of "ancestral" diets use to make.
Obviously one of the immediate benefits of intermittent fasting is the reduction of body fat, often a very important reduction, without an appreciable drop in lean mass: in fact when fasting is maintained between 16 and 24 hours in the body the fuel of choice for metabolic processes it becomes fat, with an important use of triglycerides that are recovered through mobilization of stocks of adipose tissue, while the use of proteins as a source of energy does not increase significantly until the third day of fasting. This makes it a food approach used by sportsmen and bodybuilders who want to increase muscle definition without sacrificing the much needed lean mass. [
Very interesting are studies on different animal models, from mice to monkeys, which show how caloric restriction, or intermittent fasting without an overall reduction in caloric intake, can have a protective effect against a whole series of aging-related damage , so as to increase the lifespan of people of different species, with reduced blood glucose and insulin levels and increased resistance of nervous tissue to stress damage. A possible elixir of

long life, as some enthusiastic authors affirm.

Several studies show that intermittent fasting significantly improves the blood lipid profile.

Studies based on a protocol every other day showed:

reduction of LDL cholesterol, the one commonly called "bad" cholesterol due to its possible role in the genesis of cardiovascular diseases;

reduction of triglycerides which, simplifying, we can define forms of accumulation of excess energy introduced with diet and potential risk factor as well as for cardiovascular diseases also for insulin resistance and metabolic syndrome;

a substantial maintenance of HDL cholesterol levels, the "good" cholesterol that according to some authors would have a protective effect against heart and vascular diseases.

Recent studies have shown a positive action on some markers of inflammation following fasting and even a reduction of symptoms in subjects suffering from asthma, kept for 8 weeks at a regimen with alternate days, with a marked improvement in the indicators of inflammation and stress oxidative. Another possible positive effect, highlighted in studies on animal models, is expressed on oxidative stress, synaptic plasticity and reduction of DNA damage in different brain areas, so that studies of this type are in progress to evaluate a possible use of these practices in neuro degenerative diseases characterized by chronic inflammation of the affected tissues, such as Alzheimer's disease. We are still at the beginning but the results obtained on mice are encouraging.

Many studies on intermittent fasting have been carried out on individuals who observe Ramadan, subjects who for religious reasons abstain from consuming food from dawn to dusk for a whole month. A common result was a reduction in body weight, an increase in adiponectin with a consequent increase in insulin sensitivity and therefore an improvement in glucose control: results that suggest a possible use of these practices in the prevention of type II diabetes, especially in obese or overweight subjects.

Finally, several studies on the animal model have shown a lower incidence of certain types of cancer, greater resistance after inoculation of tumor cultures and a significant reduction in the speed of proliferation of some types of cancer cells. There are still no human studies, but the results collected suggest a possible effect of intermittent fasting on some risk factors for various tumors.

Intermittent fasting is absolutely contraindicated during pregnancy and lactation, in subjects with thyroid problems, in subjects with type I or type II diabetes treated with insulin and other drugs (in the latter case medical supervision is necessary to adapt doses of the drug). And obviously it is not recommended in all subjects who suffer from eating disorders.

The name is clear. During intermittent fasting, periods are eaten when one eats during periods of fasting. It is not a real diet. Rather, a food program that tells you when - and not what - to eat.

# Chapter 2<sup>nd</sup>

## The Classic approach

When you are about to follow The Plant Paradox diet, you may advise to cut down the intake of the lectin from your diet because of its adverse health effects. In the previous chapter, you have studied the dietary guidelines and benefits of following the Plant Paradox diet. You get some knowledge about the ill effects of consuming lectin in your diet. But have you wondered that drinking a little lectin will help you in many ways? Let us discuss in this chapter the good things about lectins. But first, let me explain what lectin is exactly?

Lectin
Lectins are carbohydrate-binding proteins that are ubiquitous and mostly found in legumes and grains. These lectins bound to sugars and form glycoproteins which perform many functions like regulating the immune system. These play a role in recognition of the cellular level and molecular level.
You may also have heard that consuming too many lectins in your diet will harm you and cause nausea, muscle fatigue, cause damage to the intestine, and interferes with nutrient absorption. It is the reason why people want to eliminate the uptake of lectin. But this is not precisely something which we know about lectins.
There are always two sides of coins, and if something has a disadvantage, then there is also an advantage of that thing too. So, let us take a look at the good stuff about lectins.

The good things about lectin
- Consuming a small amount of lectin in diet sometimes helps good gut bacteria to colonize in the human digestive system and prevent adhering to pathogenic bacteria.
- Research has also shown that lectin has the potential to treat the illness caused by bacteria, fungi, and viruses. They show through the analysis that lectin is effective against several types of bacteria that cause staph infection. They also have blocked the fungal growth, which causes disease.
- Lectins are also involved in cell adhesion and are also thought to be

involved in immune function and help in the synthesis of glycoproteins.

- According to research that occurred in the 2015 review from China, published in *Cell proliferation* Proves that the lectin present in plants can help modify the expression of immune cells and also alter the cell signaling pathway to prevent the growth of cancerous cells and also block tumour growth. It can play a vital role in cancer prevention by binding to the cell membrane of cancerous cells and kill them to prevent cancer.
- The lectin shows the antimicrobial property, and in some case studies, proved that lectin serves anti-inflammatory actions.
- These are also thought to be rich in protein.

The good things about lectins show that complete elimination of this protein will not provide you any benefit. But consuming too many lectins can cause an ill effect on your health. Consume a little lectin will load you with several benefits that explained above. The food which is rich in lectin is Tomato, eggplants, beans, lentils, etc.

Some may prevent cancer by consuming lectin in their diet but have you ever discussed or wonder how alkaline stomach medium can prevent you from disease?

Coming to the next topic to show how cancer can prevent by alkaline medium

Alkaline medium and cancer prevention

The cancerous cells are thought to increase in the acidic medium and are also known to acidify their environment. But their deregulation has been observed in the person who has an alkaline stomach medium. According to a computational study done by chemist Miquel Duran-Frigola in the Institute of research Biomedicine, Barcelona shows that the cancerous cell proliferates less in the alkaline medium and in a restricted manner whose stomach pH is low. Thus, this new approach will help in finding a new way of treatment for this life-threatening disease.

A low-acid diet prevent cancer

The theories have been in concern that consuming a high-alkaline diet can help in fighting against cancer even prevent it. So, consuming right amount of food items including vegetables, fruits and eliminating acidic foods from the diet increase the pH of the blood, which creates an alkaline environment in the body that prevents cancerous cells growth.

But this is not precisely right said by Mitchell L. Gaynor, founder of Gaynor Integrative Oncology in New York in his studies *The Plan of Gene Therapy: Controlling the Genetic Destiny with Healthy Lifestyle and Good Diet*. He says that an alkaline diet help in the prevention of cancer and help in fighting cancer by controlling inflammation in the body. But they do not change the pH of the blood, and there is no role of a low acidic diet in improving the pH of the blood. Also, you can't change the pH of the stomach because your lungs and kidney will range the pH to the right amount on what you eat.

As with many dietary theories and various experiments conducted in the laboratory, proved that cancerous cells will bloom in the acidic conditions, and research shows that tumour cells are highly metabolic active and the environment around them is slightly acidic. Gaynor says, the cancerous cells also produce lactic acid through the metabolic process, which is known as the Cori cycle.

However, the theory of low acid and consuming a high-alkaline diet will help you in preventing cancer and fight against this disease. It is because the only thing to follow a healthy lifestyle is the diet. It is something that we can control. The acidity and alkalinity of food will depend upon the pH value. Alkaline foods items which includes vegetables, fruits, legumes, root vegetables, nuts are helpful in the breakdown of short-chain fatty acids which contains nutrients that will provide nourishment to the gut microbes. These bacteria, in turn, help in reducing the inflammation in your body, which might cause cancer. But the food like sugars, flour, meat, and any other animal skin can increase the acidity in the stomach and also make it difficult for the gut microbes to survive and take nutrition from the food thereby increases inflammation, said by Gaynor. Thus, a low pH diet might help fight against cancer But, there is also another theory that means that a low-acid diet will not increase your response to chemotherapy. Also, there is no need to purchase individual alkaline food products to fight for cancer.

Though Cimperman suggests that, the individual can safely have a high-alkaline diet which is suffering from cancer but only up to a limit because cancer patients are already restricted to nutrition and food intake while on treatment.

Theories may conflict, and research keeps on changing, though the evidence has provided to remove conflict from your mind about the consumption of lectin and a low-pH diet to prevent cancer. It is up to you to choose the right and guide you from the information provided in the chapter to take a healthy step for a healthy lifestyle. Keep on reading the sections, and you will find some delicious ways to enjoy your food without worrying about calories and illness.

## How it works the intermittent fast diet: possible alternatives

Food-induced thermogenesis the fundamentals of "traditional" dietetics suggest losing weight also taking advantage of the specific dynamic action of food, or energy expenditure attributable to digestive, absorption and metabolic processes.

In practice, for the same number of calories introduced, increasing the breakdown of meals makes it possible to burn more energy to process them. This makes it possible to reduce the time spans "on an empty stomach" avoiding "hunger" and keeping the metabolism fast.
Cortisol and Thyroid Hormones

Some argue that this practice also favors the containment of an unwanted hormone, cortisol (also called the "stress" hormone) and the maintenance of thyroid function (TSH and T3). Obviously, this system works as long as the caloric amount, the nutritional distribution and the glycemic load-indexes of the meals are appropriate.

### Prevent Catabolism

At the same time, in the context of muscle growth, it is (or was) a common opinion that to favor anabolism it was necessary to "feed" continuously (and "as much as possible", avoiding the adiposity increase) muscle fibrocells, in order to cancel any form of catabolism and promote proteosynthesis, ESPECIALLY thanks to insulin stimulation.
To put this food program into practice, there are several schemes

### The most popular are:
- Scheme 16:8: divides the day into two parts, with 8 hours of eating and 16 hours of fasting. It is considered an extension of the night fast: you skip breakfast and eat the first meal at noon, continuing to eat until 20.00;
- Scheme 5:2 (every other day): for 2 days a week we eat at most 500/600 kcalories. These two days must not be consecutive. In the remaining 5 you can eat whatever you want;
- Eat Stop Eat scheme: eat and fast every other day. This pattern is repeated once or twice a week.
- Scheme 5:30, is not a real fast, but the same function because for 5 days there is a very restricted hypocaloric diet to be repeated every month

In each of these schemes it is allowed to drink low-calorie beverages during the day. Water, coffee and tea without sugar are therefore allowed; milk is forbidden.

**How does it work**

In conditions of food abstinence, in addition to a total insulin calm (we recall that insulin is the anabolic hormone par excellence but also responsible for the adipose deposit) we are witnessing a significant increase in another rather "interesting" hormone: the IGF -1 or somatomedin (some also mention an increase in testosterone).
The long food deprivation is then responsible for the secretion of GH (somatotropin), also called "growth hormone" or, more sympathetically, "wellness hormone". Unlike insulin, GH, while increasing hypertrophy, does not cause adipose deposits, but the opposite! In other words, it favors the lipolysis necessary for weight loss. In practice, GH improves body composition "in the round".
For example, even in body-building, to increase muscles and decrease fat, it is essential to periodize diet and training by pursuing one and then the other goal separately; today, since intermittent fasting improves body composition bilaterally (by increasing muscle mass and losing weight), it seems to be the only true solution to all problems.

# Scheme 16:8

Dedicated to those in a hurry to make peace with the scale, it promises to lose weight quickly: it is based on the rule of 16 hours of fasting and 8 hours in which 3 meals are allowed, this diet pushes to burn fat and limits the sense of hunger , but it is not suitable for everyone.

## First application of the scheme 16:8

This protocol is made up of 3 daily meals, of which 1 snack with a fasting window of 16 hours, with or without physical activity. This is possible by combining the vegetarian-based diet with this food program.

- 1st full vegetarian or meat meal at lunchtime h. About 13.00
- 2nd meal Vegetarian-based snack h. 17.00 approx
- Preferably light physical activity (running or gymnastics) max 30 minutes after a meal or snack.
- If you love sweets you can eat them between lunch and dinner, at least 30 minutes before a physical activity
- 3rd complete meal absolutely vegetarian based at dinner time h. 20.00 approx
- Fasting window from 9.00 pm to 1.00 pm the following day (16 consecutive hours)

We remind you that you can drink low-calorie drinks throughout the day. Water, coffee and tea without sugar are therefore allowed; milk is forbidden.

At the bottom of the book you will find delicious vegetable-based recipes: a wide choice to avoid having to eat the same dishes every day and thus satisfy your hunger and allow yourself a healthy and long-lasting lifestyle

## Second Application of Scheme 16: 8

For those who do not have particular problems of excessive overweight and want to increase their muscles
I will describe below the most interesting and undoubtedly best apt variant that I believe is valid and obtains clearly visible results in the gym.
First of all I emphasize that:
although the window of fasting is exploited, the remaining meals CANNOT be consumed in freedom; moreover, to maximize the results of weight loss (and obviously those of increased muscle mass) it is always NECESSARY to perform the right physical activity.

The protocol differs in 3 daily meals and 1 training session with a fasting window of 16 hours.

- 1st meal to be consumed as soon as you get up: protein source and medium-low glycemic index carbohydrates; low fat
- 2nd meal - breakfast: complete
- Physical activity (running, weights, gymnastics)
- 3rd meal (to be carried out IMMEDIATELY after training) - lunch: complete
- Fasting window from about 13:00 or around 15:00 until the following morning.

We remind you that you can drink low-calorie drinks throughout the day. Water, coffee and tea without sugar are therefore allowed; milk is forbidden.

At the bottom of the book you will find  delicious vegetable-based recipes: a wide choice to avoid having to eat the same dishes every day and thus satisfy your hunger and allow yourself a healthy and long-lasting lifestyle

## Scheme 5:2

The 5:2 diet includes 5 days a week in which you can eat normally taking all foods without exception and two days of calorie restriction.

The two hypocaloric days must be characterized by taking a quarter of the usual caloric supply or 600 calories (250 calories for breakfast and 350 calories for dinner). Everyone is free to choose which days of the week are most convenient for fasting but it is important that these are not consecutive.

The basic principle of the 5: 2 diet is that man has developed over the millennia in conditions of caloric restriction and not in the abundance to which we are accustomed today and therefore fasting must be a favorable condition for human development. Furthermore, it has been scientifically proven that fasting makes life expectancy higher in animals.

Listening to opinions and testimonies, it would seem that this diet works, and the reasons are many! Let's try to list some of them:

Not lacking in anything: restaurant dinners, happy hours, social life

Does not make you short-tempered or depressed

It is perfect for everyone, including vegetarians

It changes the appetite and the way of eating for the benefit of physical fitness and health

It guarantees a lasting result and you don't recover the lost pounds

It loses weight without losing muscle mass

Improves health by making it more resistant to diseases such as diabetes, heart disease and some forms of cancer

It gives a feeling of general well-being: it feels more agile and energetic, the eyes and the skin become brighter

## The weekly menu 5:2

The weekly menu is another of the positive aspects of this diet, precisely the great freedom it grants to those who follow it with regards to the menu, at least in the days of regular meal which are 5 out of 7 for which you will be free to eat what you are already eating without any limitation.

Regarding the 2 days of low calorie diet, which we recommend to choose based on your daily life, a vegetarian based diet is absolutely recommended. At the bottom of the book you will find delicious vegetable-based recipes: a wide choice to avoid having to eat the same dishes every day and thus satisfy your hunger and allow yourself a healthy and long-lasting lifestyle

## Scheme Eat, Stop, Eat

The method is an alternation of whole days between fasting, low-calorie diet and classic day.

In practice for 24 hours fast (example Monday-Thursday): with possibility throughout the day to drink low-calorie beverages. Water, coffee and tea without sugar are therefore allowed; milk is forbidden.

The following 24 hours (example Tuesday-Friday): low-calorie day with a vegetarian-based diet. At the bottom of the book you will find delicious vegetable-based recipes: a wide choice to avoid having to eat the same dishes every day and thus satisfy your hunger and allow yourself a healthy and long-lasting lifestyle

The following 24 hours (example Wednesday-Saturday): normal day you can eat whatever you want, but in moderation.

For those who want to get results in a short time we start again for the second time with the same technique in order to complete the week.

The extra day usually on Sundays there is no food limitation

For all the others they can start again from the following Monday with fasting-low-calorie-normal food

A light physical activity during the day in which you will do the normal day is however recommended to improve skin firming, in view of weight reduction.

## Scheme 5:30

The "5:30" diet also makes it possible to slow aging. Confirmation would come from a trial conducted on 100 individuals.

The type of power supply

The research started in order to understand the effects of this type of diet in the prevention of diseases associated with aging. People aged 20-70 years, some overweight or obese, were involved, who for three months for five days each month followed a diet that included 800-1100 calories a day (low calorie diet) with low sugar and protein, but rich in unsaturated fats, the good ones (which we find for example in fish or extra virgin olive oil). It included tea, energy bars, small snacks and vegetable-based foods

## Reduction of risk factors

It has emerged that following the aforementioned dietary regime the risk factors for diabetes, cancer and cardiovascular diseases are reduced, including the reduction of abdominal fat (the "bad" accumulated on the stomach), blood pressure, cholesterol, and factor inflammatory CRP, of the IGF-1 molecule associated with cancer and aging, all without loss of muscle mass (one of the dangers of excessively strict diets or real fasts).

Why eat a little while ago "rejuvenate"

Another study published in the journal Molecular & Cellular Proteomics clarifies better how eating little affects cell aging. The researchers tested the calorie restriction on a group of mice and found that their protein production slowed down. The proteins are synthesized by the "ribosomes": when the ribosomes have "stopped" they have had time to repair themselves, in simple terms of "rejuvenating". "The ribosome is a very complex machine and a bit like your car needs periodic maintenance to replace the parts that wear out the fastest," explained John Price, professor of biochemistry at Brigham Young University and lead author of the study . «When the tires wear out, the whole car is not thrown away. It is more convenient to replace the tires ». Mice on a low-calorie diet were more energetic and suffered from fewer diseases, "said Price. "And not only did they live longer, they kept their bodies better and stayed young longer."

### BENEFITS of the intermittent diet

In recent years, any diet that includes periods of fasting or caloric restriction is considered "anti-aging": precisely called intermittent fasting, which can be followed in different ways that adapt to each type of person. The benefits of this practice so simple to adopt are based on scientific studies and evidences now widely shared: fasting improves health in general and prolongs life expectancy due to its effects on the functioning of cells and hormones. It is sufficient to abstain from food for 24 hours, for example, because new neurons are formed in the brain and our body becomes "defensive" by adopting a series of "virtuous" precautions: lowering inflammation, improving the immune response and enhancing capacity of cells to get rid of waste substances. Not only that, caloric abstention even slows down the growth of tumors, at least in mice, as shown by a detailed article published in Proceedings of the National Academy of Sciences, which puts together all the advantages of this food practice.

## How to put it into practice

The 5:30 scheme is an entirely vegetable low-calorie food protocol.
It lasts 5 days and includes 1150 kcal on the 1st day and approximately 800 kcal from the 2nd to the 5th day.

At the bottom of the book you will find  delicious vegetable-based recipes: a wide choice to avoid having to eat the same dishes every day and thus satisfy your hunger and allow yourself a healthy and long-lasting lifestyle.

You will feel hungry during these 5 days, but the purpose is precisely this: to make the brain understand that it must optimize all the functions of the body, expel cells that are no longer efficient, improve and rejuvenate those that can be recovered, burn fat on access, reduce inflammation of organs.
This, finding itself in a condition of controlled caloric restriction, behaves as if it were fasting and starts a process of cell renewal, with which it eliminates what is no longer necessary and replaces it with new and healthy cells.

## ASSESSED BENEFITS

- Activates stem cell-based renewal in the body for anti-aging benefits
- Lose weight and reduce abdominal fat for better health
- Extend your healthy life with simple daily changes
- Prevents bone and muscle loss
- Build your resistance to diabetes, cardiovascular disease, Alzheimer's disease and cancer

# Chapter 4$^{th}$

## "Regenerative medicine" for cell health

Man lives, breathes and is able to cure himself in different ways. Nothing is
more representative of this process of cell regeneration and regenerative
medicine. But what is "regenerative medicine"?
For example, when you cut yourself, you heal and the wound disappears after
about a week: this is the regeneration of epithelial cells.
The berries help build the powerful antioxidant superoxide dismutase (SOD),
excellent for reducing oxidative stress: a key factor in liver support and in
preventing joint pain.
Each individual has the ability to regenerate their cells: it is programmed for
this, and that is how it grows, develops and heals. For example, when you cut
yourself, you heal and the wound disappears after about a week: this is the
regeneration of epithelial cells.
Bones and ligaments are also living matter that breathes. Each single cell of
the human skeleton is replaced every seven years. However, the human being
does not have the ability to self-recreate a leg or an arm, as well as many other
tissues (a young salamander, on the other hand, can regenerate its paw
completely in about five weeks).
A primary objective of regenerative medicine is therefore to find ways to
trigger tissue regeneration in the human body or to form replacement tissues.

Scientists, doctors and futurists around the world, in fact, assert that the
future of medicine lies in understanding how the body develops from a single
cell and the mechanisms it uses to renew itself throughout life. In this way it
will be possible to replace damaged tissues and intervene to help the body
regenerate: there is therefore the potential to cure or alleviate the symptoms
of people with disorders such as heart disease, Alzheimer's, Parkinson's,
diabetes, spinal cord injury and tumors.
Currently, from stem cell researchers (adult cells that can develop into many
different types of tissues) that study to induce the body to heal itself, positive
results have been found in the treatment of congestive heart failure and in
muscle regrowth in wounded soldiers in explosions.

## CELL REGENERATION - WHICH BODIES CAN BE REGENERATED?

There is a wide range of stem cell-based therapies today. The scientists created tissue patches for burn victims; furthermore, since diabetics suffer from damage to beta cells, the regeneration of these cells has become a point of maximum attention, and scientists have developed so-called 'pancreatic islands' (groups of cells that produce insulin) to treat diabetes by transplanting them by the hundreds.

Due to Alzheimer's and dementia, the regeneration of brain cells has become another primary goal. Scientists have also developed healthy brain cells to alleviate symptoms caused by diseases such as Parkinson's disease, and have been able to genetically modify cells, using them to provide healing or protection to injured or diseased areas of the body.

An international team of researchers and collaborators from the US clinic, Mayo, for example, has discovered a way to regenerate heart tissue: using stem cell therapy instead of drugs to manage heart damage, the heart can indeed repair itself. Stem cells are collected from a patient's bone marrow and subjected to a laboratory treatment that causes them to turn into cardiac cells, which are then injected into the patient's heart to develop healthy cardiac tissues.

Ginger combats painful inflammation by inhibiting the effects of arachidonic acid, a necessary fat that causes the inflammatory response

There are other similar therapies for the regeneration of the spinal cord, the cartilage of the knee and the hip, for the repair of the tooth and gums, the eyes and even the brain. And finally, the kidneys: researchers at the Stanford Institute for Stem Cell Biology and Regenerative Medicine and Sheba Medical Center and Sackler Medical School in Israel recently revealed how the kidneys grow steadily and have a surprising ability to regenerate - overturning the consolidated idea that this was impossible - by opening a path towards new ways of healing and also re-growing the kidneys.

Also the liver, in this sense, is among all the organs of the body of extreme importance, as it is endowed with the maximum regenerative capacity: after injuries or illnesses, the liver can recreate itself in order to continue to perform an adequate function, even if it does not return to its original form.

When, however, the liver is damaged beyond its own capacity for regeneration, transplantation is achieved, the waiting lists can be long; so transplant surgeons and other researchers are developing regenerative therapies based on liver cells.

A primary objective of regenerative medicine is therefore to find ways to trigger tissue regeneration in the human body or to form replacement tissues.

## CELL REGENERATION - RISK FACTORS

There are concerns about cell regeneration, if it does not occur naturally, so it is preferable to use a food program, rather than medicine at present because despite the clinical potential, there are also potential and unexpected risks. An invitation to assess any potential risks should always be an indispensable prerequisite before clinically using a therapy or stem cell-based medicines.

The risks, according to the Journal of Translational Medicine, depend on the type of stem cells used, the way they are administered to the body, where they are applied, the phases of manipulation (are they embryonic cells or adult stem cells?), and are related to the irreversibility of the treatment, the need for tissue regeneration in the event of an irreversible tissue loss and the long-term survival of the implanted cells.

The risks identified from clinical experience or the potential risks observed in animal studies include tumor formation, unwanted immune responses and infections.

Serious side effects have been reported in some clinical studies, highlighting the need for further experiments. It is still a young science: the knowledge of its safety and its long-term efficacy are partial.

For this reason it is better to create a regenerative environment using a food program that allows to achieve the same result, but in a completely natural way

## THE SIX BEST REGENERATIVE CELLS FOR CELLS

Diet plays an important role in the regeneration cycles of the human body. This is because food choices are like building materials, on which availability will depend the quality of the new replacement cells that will be built. It is reasonable, therefore, that by eating the right foods, the newly formed cells can be stronger and healthier than the ones they will replace.

It is well known: inflammation is the body's response to injury, infection, irritation or imbalance. Eating anti-inflammatory foods can be a valuable aid in protecting and regenerating your cells. What does an anti-inflammatory diet include? The abolition of fried and processed foods, the introduction of fresh whole foods containing phytonutrients and a vegetable-based diet.

The following are the six main foods recommended to help general cell regeneration:

1. Forest fruits. Blueberries, raspberries, blackberries help build the powerful antioxidant superoxide dismutase (SOD), excellent for reducing oxidative stress: a key factor for liver support and joint pain prevention. The berries are also rich in flavonoids which reduce inflammation and repair cellular damage.

2. Broccoli. Broccoli may not be preferred by children, but this cruciferous vegetable is rich in sulforapan, a chemical that increases enzymes in the liver, which work to neutralize the harmful toxins we breathe. Furthermore, all cruciferous vegetables have a molecule called indole-3-carbinol which reduces inflammatory agents in the blood.

3. Ginger root. Ginger root, in addition to solving stomach problems, fights painful inflammations by inhibiting the effects of arachidonic acid, the necessary fat that triggers the inflammatory response.

4. Walnuts and seeds. These practical snacks have healthy fats and proteins to satiate you for a long time and satisfy your cravings; but their benefits do not end there: walnuts like hazelnuts, almonds and seeds like those of flax, hemp and chia contain a lot of alpha-linolenic acid, a type of anti-inflammatory omega-3 fat. The seeds also contain plant sterols, also known for their anti-inflammatory properties.

5. Mushrooms, which have always been a mainstay in traditional medicine, such as shiitake and maiitake are rich in polyphenols. These are nutrients known to help protect liver cells from damage. Supporting the liver is essential in the fight against inflammation, as it filters toxins and breaks down hormones.

6. Fatty fish and seafood. Seafood contains eicosapentaenoic acid, an omega-3 fatty acid that is a powerful anti-inflammatory. Several studies show that the oil contained in the fish can act as an anti-inflammatory.

A plant-based diet is in itself a good anti-inflammatory; if we add to this an intermittent feeding program the result is the return to its own weight (weight under control as from young), improvement of health, delay of aging, natural acceleration of metabolism, natural cell renewal. In practice, feeling young and in full force even if you are no longer 20 years old.

# Chapter 5<sup>th</sup>

**The top delicious vegetarian  recipes for beginners**

In this chapter we are going to give you a brief of top  delicious  vegetarian recipes that you could enjoy without thinking about your calorie count and nutritional level. These recipes are rich in essential nutrients, healthy fats, and good cholesterol which will give your body of healthy life. We have not limited to only the main meal recipes but keeping your all cravings in mind we provided a complete package of recipe which includes everything starting from your breakfast, lunch and dinner. The list does not just end here as we also keep in mind about your snack cravings and yes deserts, which everybody loves. So, let us start with the delicious smoothies' recipes which you enjoy in your breakfast.

## Smoothies

The smoothies give you perfect start for a day. Not only these smoothies fill up your stomach but also load you with antioxidants, healthy carbs and fats. It gives a protein kick to start your day and lose fat easily. Let us take a look at different smoothie recipe which you can enjoy within minutes without hurdles.

# 1. Blueberry Beet smoothie

This delicious smoothie combines with the goodness of berries and beetroot full of nutrition. It is loaded with protein and omega -3 fatty acids with vitamins, minerals, and fibre.

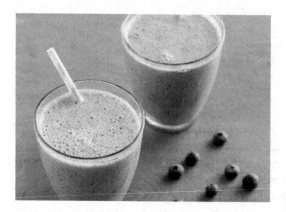

## Ingredients:

- half cup blueberries
- half cup banana
- one small peeled tangerine
- one tablespoon chia seed optional
- one fourth teaspoon cinnamon
- one fourth cup yogurt (fat-free)
- one beetroot sliced and peeled
- Ice

## Method:

Put the ingredients listed above into mixer grinder jar and grind it until thick paste. serve It in breakfast even lunch and dinner.

## Nutrition:

Total calories: 287 calories
Protein content: 18gms
Carbohydrates: 50gms
Fat: 4gms
Fibres- 10gm

## 2. The purple smoothie (lectin-free)

**Total time to prepare:** 5 min

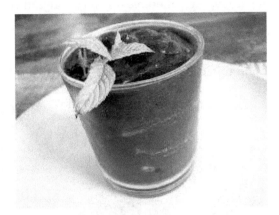

**Ingredients:** ¼ cup of almond milk or you can also use coconut milk

1 handful spinach
¼ cup sweet potato (purple)
¼ cup yogurt
1 cup berries
1 drop liquid stevia

**Instructions:** Put all the ingredients in the blender that are listed above and blend until a smooth consistency is formed.

Serve it and enjoy it.

**Nutrition:**

Calories: 61

Protein: 2 g

Fat: 1.3 g

Cholesterol: 0.0 mg

Vitamin A: 17%

### 3. Keto beetroot smoothie

The keto beetroot smoothie gives you a healthy kick of antioxidants and builds immunity in you. This smoothie is rich in fibre and vitamin C. It gives you a perfect start for the day. Let us take a look at how you can prepare this delicious recipe.

**Total preparation time:** 7 min

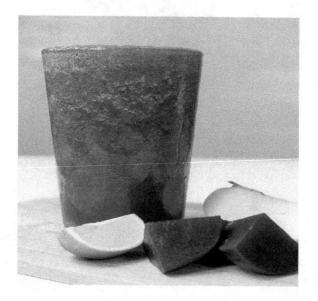

**Ingredients:** 2 beetroots boiled

1 raw celery stalk

½ cup cucumber chopped

1 teaspoon coconut oil

½ cup almond milk

**Instructions to cook:** Chop all the above listed ingredients. Put all of them in blender. Add almond milk and coconut oil and blend to make a smooth consistency

Serve into the glass with ice
**Nutrition:** Calorie: 300
Fat: 20g
Carbohydrates: 6g
Fibre: 3g
Protein: 25g
Vitamin C: 60%

## 4. The detox green smoothie

This detox green smoothie helps you eliminating harmful toxins from the body. This smoothie helps you in filling your stomach with right nutrition and is perfect for breakfast.

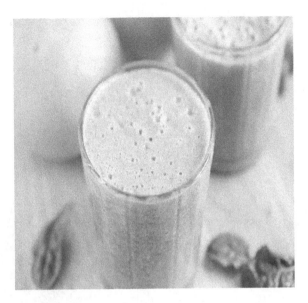

**Total Cooking time:** 5 min

**Ingredients:** 1 cup chopped green lettuce, ½ cup mint leaves, ½ cup spinach, ½ cup avocado, 3 tablespoon lemon juice, 3 drops stevia extract, 1 cup water.

**Cooking instructions:** Simply put all the ingredients into the blender and blend them to form a smooth consistency. Serve it by putting ice in it.

**Nutrition:** Calorie: 280

Fat: 20g

Carbohydrates: 14 g

Fibre: 10g

Protein: 15g

## 5. The hemp seed protein smoothie

This hemp protein smoothie loads you with protein and healthy carbs so that you can start your day with healthy nutrition.

**Total cooking time:** 7 min

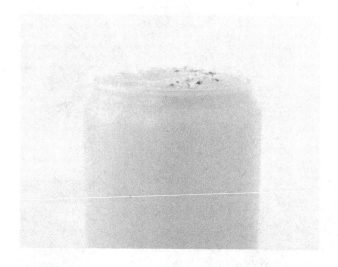

**Ingredients:** 2 cups spinach, 1cup kale leaves, 2 tablespoon hemp protein, 2 drops of liquid stevia, ice cubes, 2 cup water.

**Cooking instructions:** Put the ingredients into the blender. Blend the mixture on high power for few seconds. Now put some ice cubes into the glass. Pour the smoothie and enjoy it.

**Nutrition:** Calorie: 250

Fat: 10g

Protein: 7 g

Carbohydrate: 35 g

Fibre: 9g

## 6. Kiwifruit smoothie recipe with honeydew melon

This sweet delicious tangy, sweet, green smoothie is good for health and has anti-inflammatory properties. This smoothie is rich in calcium, with a dose of protein, fibre, vitamins A, C.

**Total preparation time:** 5 min

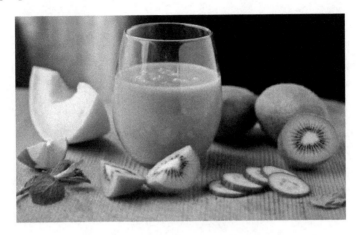

**Ingredients:**

- One cup melon chopped
- Half cup yogurt
- Half cup fat-free milk
- One spoon honey
- Half teaspoon cinnamon
- One and a half cup kiwifruit, peeled

**Method:**

Put all the ingredients in the jug grind to make a smooth paste and serve it.

**Nutrition:**
Calories: 285
Protein: 18gm
Carbohydrates: 50gm
Fibre: 5gm
Fat: 1.5gm

## 7. Apple, spinach smoothie

This green smoothie is sweet and delicious. It is loaded with proteins, Vitamins, and dietary fibre. It helps you in weight management and provides various health benefits and maintain good cholesterol in you.

**The preparation time:** 7 min

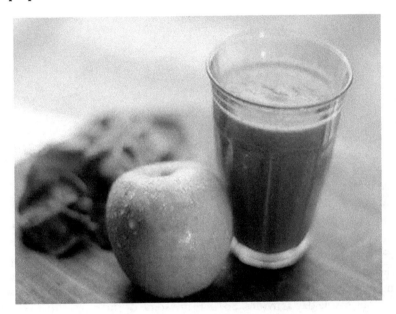

**Ingredients:**

One medium-size apple sliced

One spoon lime juice

One tangerine sliced peeled

Half tablespoon ginger chopped

One cup blanched spinach leaf

One cup of yogurt

One spoon honey

Crushed ice

**Method**

Put all the chopped ingredients in the grinder jar and grind it till a smooth paste informed. Serve it fresh.

**Nutrition:**

Calories: 246

Protein: 15gm

Carbohydrates: 50gm

Fat: 1 gm

Fibre: 5 gm

**Breakfast Salads, main course and side dishes**

When we talk about the main dishes, our stomach not only fills with food but with the right type of food. Here we have provided the best recipes which you can enjoy in your breakfast, lunch and dinner. We have detailed a complete package of recipes with their cooking time and nutrient values. Your breakfast and main dish should be loaded with essential nutrients to keep you energise for your whole day activities. So, here are some of the recipes that you can enjoy in your day.

## 8. Broccoli pesto cilantro salad

This salad serves as the best option for detoxing your body. This is because it consists of ingredients like garlic, cilantro, and broccoli which act as detoxifiers and also helps in detoxifying the liver, digestive system, and kidney.

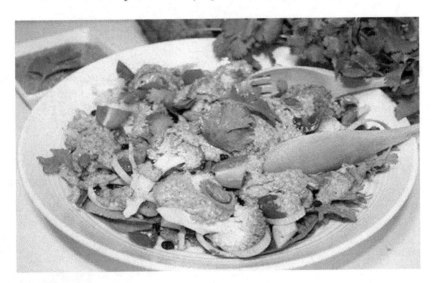

**Cooking time:** 25 min

### Ingredients:

- Two cups green leafy vegetable kale, spinach, lettuce
- One cup Broccoli chopped
- Half cup leek sliced
- 200 gm cherry tomatoes
- One avocado chopped
- One fourth cup Pistachios nuts
- One fourth cup coriander stems (optional)

### For dressings

One cup coriander leaf for garnishing

125ml olive oil

Garlic crushed

Lemon juice

Table salt

Black pepper as per your taste

One lime, optional

**Method:**

Steam the broccoli for 2 mins. Prepare salad ingredients chopped them and put them into the bowl. Pour all the ingredients and broccoli and process them into a blender. Garnish with fresh coriander leaves chopped.

**Nutrition:**

Calories: 300 per serving

Sodium: 50mg

Carbohydrates: 17gm

Fibre: 6gm

Fat: 25gm

Protein: 7gm

## 9. Mexican corn and black bean lettuce wraps

This vegan spin Mexican wrap is delicious with a dose of healthy fruits and vegetables. This crunchy lettuce is perfect for satisfying protein needs and provides you ample of antioxidants. The guacamole healthy monounsaturated fats allow your body to absorb nutrients from the vegetables. It can serve with rice and grilled vegetables.

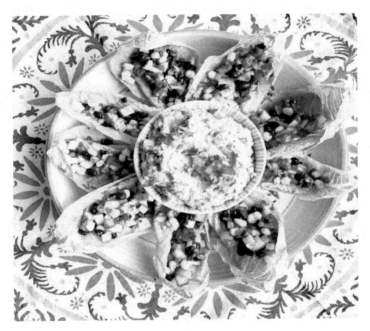

**Cooking time:** 30 min

**Ingredients:**

One cup corn kernel

One cup chopped onions

One cucumber chopped

One can beans

One diced tomato

2 tablespoon chopped cilantro

Lemon zest and juice of one lemon

One to two head lettuce

Guacamole

### Guacamole preparation

Mash two ripe avocados and add 2 tablespoons chopped coriander. Now add a pinch of salt, black pepper and lime juice in it.

### Method

Put beans, corn, onion, tomato, coriander, kernels, lemon zest, and juice in a bowl. Cut some lettuce leaves and arrange them around the guacamole and filled the lettuce with mixed ingredients and garnish with cilantro. Serve it in breakfast lunch dinner.

### Nutrition:

Calories: 286

Fat: 17.4gm

Cholesterol: 0.00mg

Carbohydrates: 24gm

Fibre: 12gm

Protein: 15.1gm

Vitamin A: 74.6%

# 10. Broccoli vegan salad

A quick and delicious broccoli vegan salad recipe which is served as a side dish is rich in protein, low in carbs, loaded with veggies. One cup of broccoli can complete your daily need of vitamin C and K. Broccoli is considered as an anti-inflammatory substance, supports body detoxification, and cancer prevention. One should include it in their daily diet. Let's take a look at how you can prepare it to eat.

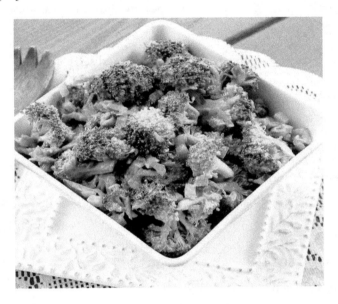

**Cooking time:** 20-25 min

**Ingredients:**

- 2-3 cups of broccoli bunch
- 1 tablespoon sesame seeds
- 1 spoon olive oil
- 3 tablespoon peanuts
- 2-3 chopped spring onions
- water as per need
- salt and black pepper to taste
- soya sauce
- chili sauce
- lemon

**Method to cook:**

Cut broccoli into small pieces and take a pan to medium heat put one spoon olive oil add broccoli to it and fry it for two minutes.

Now add some water and sauté it for 3-4 minutes. Put some soya sauce, spring onions and add sesame seeds, peanuts into it and stir it for few minutes.

Now add salt, black pepper, lemon juice in it and serve it into the bowl.

**Nutrient:**

Calorie: 200.1gm

Fats: 9.2gm

cholesterol: 3.8gm

carbohydrate: 25gm

proteins: 5.1gm

dietary fibre: 5gm

sodium: 113.1 gm

Vitamin A: 47g

## 11. Broccoli soup

The broccoli soup is filled with antioxidants and essential nutrients that keep your body healthy. The broccoli proves to be the best food which is rich in protein and healthy carbs. It loads you with perfect and balance nutrition.

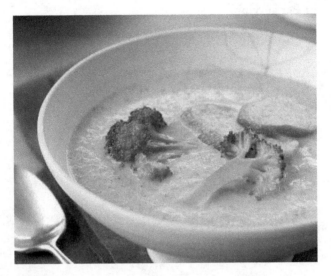

**Cooking time:** 30 min

**Ingredients:**

- 1 medium-size onion finely chopped
- extra-virgin olive oil 1 tablespoon
- 1 celery stalk freshly chopped
- 2-3 cloves garlic
- 7-8 cups chopped broccoli
- 2-3 cups water
- 3 cups vegetable broth or chicken broth
- salt
- Black pepper

**Method:**

In a pan heat extra-virgin olive oil and put onions, celery stalk, garlic clove into the oil to stir fry. Fry till the raw smell is gone.

Now add broccoli into it and fry it till soften. Add some vegetable broth into it and bring it to boil.

Add salt according to taste.

once the veggies are done cooled it slightly and then blend it.

Sieve the puree and boil it for 3- 4min add some salt and pepper and boil it.

serve it hot in dinner, lunch

**Nutrition: Per serving**

calories: 160,

fat: 8gm,

fibre: 5.2 gm,

carbohydrate: 17gm,

protein: 10gm,

cholestero: 17 mg,

Vitamin C 58%,

calcium 80mg,

iron 2.5mg.

## 12. The lectin-free, paleo spanakopita omelette recipe

The quick, healthy omelette recipe that gives you a perfect start for the day! It loads you with protein and omega-3-fatty acids. This omelette proves to be the perfect breakfast. One must include in their breakfast daily.

**Total cooking time:** 10 minutes

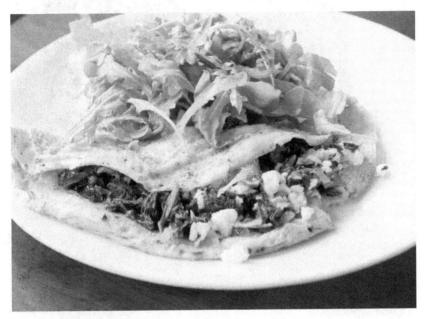

**Cooking ingredients:** 1 clove minced garlic, 1 ½ cup spinach finely chopped, 1 tablespoon butter, ¼ cup of onion, parsley 1 cup finely chopped, 1 teaspoon oregano, 2 eggs, salt, black pepper according to taste, feta cheese 1 tablespoon (optional), 1 cup arugula, extra-virgin olive oil.

**Cooking instructions:** Take butter in a pan and heat it on medium flame. Now add minced garlic and onion and stir fry till translucent.

Now add spinach, parsley, oregano into it and cook till spinach got wilted for about 3-4 min. Mix salt and pepper into it. Once it did keep these veggies aside.

In the same pan heat butter, whisk 2 eggs by adding salt and pepper and spread it into the pan to make an omelette. Once it is done remove it from the pan into the plate and serve by topping it with veggies mixture. You can also sprinkle cheese on it.

**Nutrition:** per serving

Calories: 230

Carbohydrates: 6g

Cholesterol: 2mg

Protein: 8.2gm

Fibre: 3.2gm

## 13. The sunchoke breakfast skillet

**Total cooking time:** 15-20 min

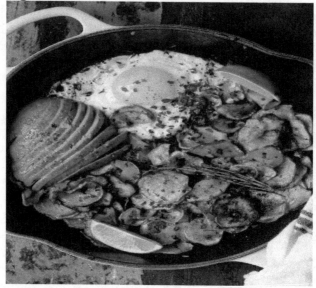

**Ingredients:** Avocado oil or ghee
1 avocado
3 medium sunchokes
One egg
Parsley
1 lime
Thyme (optional)

**Cooking Instructions:** Cut all the sunchokes and remove black spots from the surface.
Now slice them with a knife.
Now take a pan and heat oil in it.
Once oil is heated put all the sunchokes, thyme and cook it by stirring occasionally for about 10 minutes. When they are done keep it aside in the pan and pour a tablespoon of ghee in the pan space. Now break an egg into it and cook it for few minutes. Sprinkle a pinch of salt. Add parsley into it for garnishing. Now add avocado and lime and serve in a bowl or straight in the pan.

**Nutrition: Per serving**
Calorie: 280
Carbohydrate: 25g
Protein: 4g
Fibre: 3g
Fat: 5.5g

## 14. keto-friendly Almond flour pancakes

The almonds are considered to be the healthiest nuts for health. The almond pancake is keto-friendly and very easy to cook. Let us take a look at the ingredients and cooking procedure and how much nutrition it will add to you.

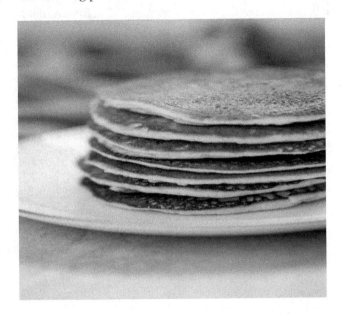

**Ingredients:**

- One cup blanched almond flour
- 1-2 eggs (for vegans you can use bananas instead of eggs)
- 2 tablespoon maple syrup or use water instead
- One teaspoon baking powder
- One tablespoon olive oil
- Salt to taste

**Cooking steps**

Stir together all ingredients almond flour, eggs, maple syrup or water, baking powder, olive oil and vanilla (optional) in a bowl to make a thick smooth batter. make sure that there are no lumps in the batter

Grease the heated pan with olive oil and pour some batter into the centre and spread it with the spoon to form a circle with little thick layer say around half an inch.

Cook until bubbles start appearing and it is fluffy. Flip it with a spatula to cook it from another side too. Serve warm with your favourite toppings in breakfast.

You can also cook in the oven all you need is to just preheat the oven and place the batter bowl in the oven to cook at 350°F for ten minutes

**Nutrition:**
Calories: 175
Fat: 15gm
Carbohydrate: 3-4 gm
Fibre: 1gm
Protein: 6gm
 1/4 teaspoon fine sea salt

## 15. Chicken with arugula salad and lemon

This is also another healthy option for the keto diet. It loads you with good carb, protein, and vitamins. Let's take a look at how you can cook it and what ingredient you need for this.

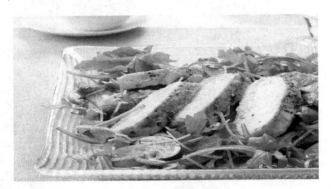

**Ingredients:**

Avocado oil
Boneless chicken 3 ounce
Lemon zest of one lemon and lemon juice
Table salt to taste
Olive oil for dressing
Freshly squeezed lemon juice
One cup arugula
Sautéed mushrooms (optional)

**Method:**

Heat the avocado oil in a pan and place chicken strips in it sprinkle salt and lemon on it and sauté for about 3 minutes till it cooks and turns it to another side so that both sides were cooked properly.
Mix lemon zest, and juice with olive oil until it mixes properly.
Slightly toss the arugula in the dressing and top up with chicken.

**For vegans:** replace chicken with tofu or a cauliflower

**Nutrients:**
Calorie: 250
Fat: 12gm
Protein: 13gm
Cholesterol: 20gm
Vitamin A: 61%
Vitamin C: 70%

## 16. Lemony brussels sprouts with cabbage, kale, and onion

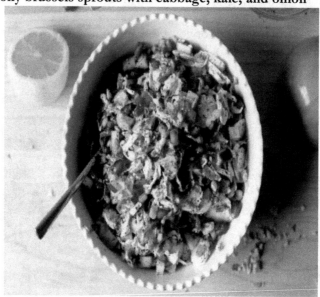

**Total time for meal:** 15-20 min

**Serving:** 1-2

**Ingredients:** One-inch thick-sliced cabbage, 1 spoon extra virgin olive oil, 4 tablespoons avocado oil, half cup thinly sliced onions, one cup brussels sprouts thin-sliced, half to one cup chopped kale, freshly squeezed lemon juice 1 spoon, salt, black pepper for taste.

**Method:**
Heat the pan and put one tablespoon avocado oil in it. Reduce the flame and add cabbage into the oil and stir fry till it turns golden brown. Add a pinch of salt and keep it into the plate aside.
Clean out the pan and add another tablespoon of avocado oil in it. Now put some sliced onions and brussels sprouts into the pan and stir it till it becomes tender soft for 3 to 4 minutes. Now add remaining avocado oil in a pan and add kale and lemon juice into it
Serve by topping the cabbage steaks with these sautéed vegetables and add some olive oil if required.

**Nutrition:**
calories: 222
Fat: 18 gm
Carbohydrates: 15gm
Fibre: 3 gm
Protein: 10gm

## 17. Sautéed cabbage-kale with Avocado and tofu

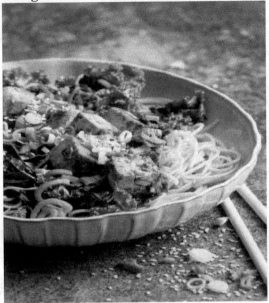

**Total time for meal cooking:** 15-20 min

**Serving:** 1-2

**Ingredients:** ½ diced Avocado, 3 tablespoon avocado oil, 1 or ½ cup cabbage finely sliced, ½ cup chopped kale, ½ cup chopped onions, 3 ounces hemp tofu, 2 tablespoon lemon juice, salt, pepper.

**Method:** Sauté avocado in lemon juice, add a pinch of salt and keep it aside. Now heat the pan and add 2 tablespoons of avocado oil into it. Now toss kale cabbage and onion into the oil till it becomes softer, continue it till 8-10 mins. Add some salt into it according to the taste.
Add the remaining avocado oil into the pan and fry to hemp tofu till it becomes softer and add lemon juice into it and sauté for about 6 minutes till both sides fried.
Serve it by adding salt and cabbage, kale avocado over it.

**Nutrition:**
Calorie: 198
Fats: 12.4 gm
Carbohydrate: 18.3 gm
Fibre: 7gm

## 18. The cauliflower rice with roasted Broccoli and sautéed onions

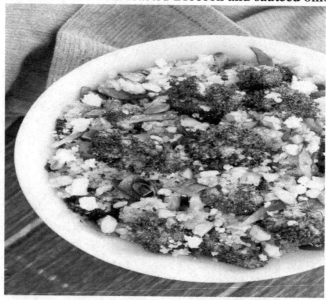

**Total time for meal preparation:** 20 minutes

**Ingredients:** half cabbage shredded in the form of rice, 4 tablespoon avocado oil, 1 teaspoon curry leaves, salt, Broccoli one cup, 1 onion chopped.

**Method:** Heat the pan and sautéed cauliflower into the avocado oil for 3 to 5 minutes. Then add lemon juice, curry leaves, and curry powder and mix them well.
Now take a pan and put some avocado oil in it and toss the broccoli into it for 5 to 10 minutes till it becomes soft and salt and lime juice into it.
Now re-heat the pan and add some onions to stir fry in the avocado oil till it becomes softer. Add some lemon juice into it. While serving the cabbage rice on a plate, add it by serving broccoli and onions sautéed on it.

**Nutrition:**

Calorie: 91

Carbohydrates: 4 gm

Protein: 3 gm

Fat: 8 gm

## 19. Carrot muffins

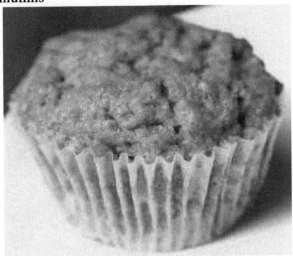

**Total time to prep meals:** 20-25 minutes

**Ingredients:** 2 grated carrots, one cup blanched almond flour, baking soda ½ teaspoon, salt 1/8th teaspoon, ½ teaspoon cinnamon, 2 cups coconut flour, nutmeg ½ teaspoon, 2 spoon yogurt, 1 spoon avocado oil, coconut milk, 2 teaspoon vanilla essence. ½ cup chopped walnuts

**Method:** Preheat the oven to 350°F. Now prepare the muffin tin cupcakes liner and keep it aside.
Take a bowl, put coconut flour, salt, the almond flour, baking soda, cinnamon, and nutmeg and whisk it gently.
In another bowl mix yogurt, oil, and coconut milk and vanilla.
Mix both mixtures and add grated carrots and walnuts. Hold the mixtures into muffin tins and bake it for 12 to 18 minutes. After baking is done, take out the muffins and keep it in an airtight container and serve it. You can keep it for about one long as well.

### Nutrition:

Calorie: 279,

fat: 16gm,

carbohydrate: 31 gm,

protein: 5%,

Vitamin A: 49%

## 20. Cheesy Brazilian bread

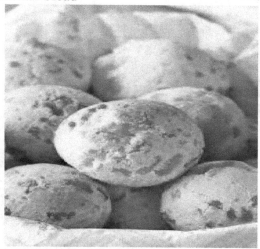

**Cooking time:** 30 minutes

**Ingredients:** One cup milk, coconut milk, condensed milk, ½ cup avocado oil, 1 teaspoon salt, 2 cups cassava flour, 2 eggs, half cup grated Parmigiano-Reggiano cheese, 1 spoon nutritional yeast.

### Directions for cooking:

Preheat microwave oven at 375°F. Now put two baking sheets along with parchment paper.

Put milk, oil, and salt in a pan. Bring it to medium heat and stir it occasionally. Remove it from heat after the boil.

Now add slowly the cassava flour into the milk and stir it continuously to avoid lump formation in them. Now transfer the dough into the bowl and beat the mixture till it becomes smooth. Put some yogurt into it and beat it till it is fully incorporated into the mixture.

Now add cheese into the mixture and scoop it out, place the scooped mixture on baking sheet and bake for 15 minutes till they bake and their colour turns into golden.

Now bring it out from the oven cool it down and serve it.

### Nutrition:

Calorie: 131.8,

carbohydrate: 13.9 gm,

protein: 3gm,

fat: 8gm

## 21. Low carb mushroom soup

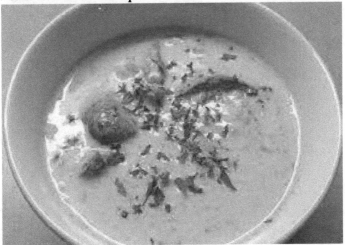

This low carb mushroom soup is perfect for those who follow a keto diet for a healthy lifestyle.

**Total time to prepare:** 45 minutes

**Ingredients:** 2 spoon butter, 4-5 cups mushrooms roughly chopped, ½ cup chopped onions, one clove garlic, salt, ½ teaspoon black pepper, vegetable broth one cup, one cup whipped cream, 1 tablespoon sherry.

**Directions to cook:** Take a saucepan heat it on medium flame. Now add butter in it. Put mushrooms, onions, garlic and cook them for few minutes or until they get soft and tender. Once mushrooms are done add salt, pepper. Cook and stir for about one minute so that all ingredients combine perfectly. Now add vegetable broth and cream into it. Reduce heat and pour it into the sherry. Blend the mixture and sieve it and serve it.

**Nutrition:**

Calorie: 440 calories,

fat: 45gm,

carbohydrates: 8 gm,

Protein: 6gm,

cholesterol: 152mg.

### 22. Spinach Cauliflower Risotto

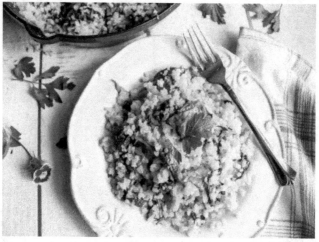

**Total time to cook:** 15 minutes

**Ingredients:** Olive oil 2 tablespoons, 2 cloves garlic cloves, One cup rice cauliflower, ½ tablespoon salt, 2 cup spinach, one fourth freshly chopped parsley,

**Cooking instruction:** Put some butter in pan, add some minced garlic and toss them for few minutes.

Once it has done Put riced cauliflower and sprinkles with salt and black pepper.

Mix it with garlic butter and allow the riced cauliflower to cook slowly and stir it till soft.

Now add spinach to it and mix it well again and cook for about 2 minutes until the spinach wilted.

After it is done, garnish with freshly chopped parsley and serve it warm.

**Nutrition:**

Calorie: 70

Fat: 11%

Protein: 14gm

Calcium: 20gm

Carbohydrates: 1g

## 23. Cream celery soup

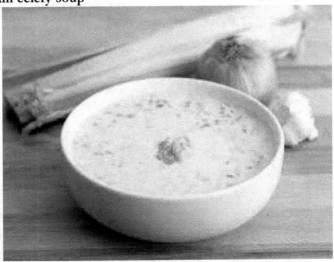

**Cook time:** 50-60 min

**Ingredients:** 1 bunch of celery roughly diced, 2 roughly diced onions, ½ garlic bulb minced, 4 cups vegetable stock, ½ cup cream, salt, black pepper, 2 bay leaves, extra-virgin olive oil, 1 avocado.

**Directions to cook:** Wash and chopped celery, onion and garlic. Heat olive oil in the pan, add cumin, celery, onion, garlic, and avocado into the oil and stir it for few minutes or till they get soft. Sauté the ingredients till they turn in light brown colour. Now add broth and cover it to boil. Keep the flame on medium.

Now remove from heat and add soup to a blender. Sieve it, add salt and black pepper and serve it and enjoy it.

**Nutrition:**

Calories: 325

Fat: 25gm

Protein: 5 gm

Carbohydrate: 12gm

## 24. Mashed cauliflower

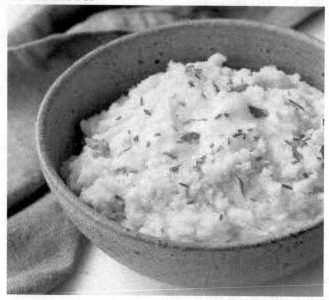

**Cooking time:** 30 min

**Ingredients:** One cauliflower head, two tablespoon butter, salt, 3-4 garlic cloves, black pepper, and coriander leaves for garnishing.

**Cooking instructions:**

Cut the cauliflower into florets and boil it in salty water for a couple of minutes or till it becomes softer. Strain the water from the cauliflower and add it to a processor with the remaining ingredients. Blend it to a thick consistency.

Pour this into the plate add a pinch of salt and pepper for taste

Garnish it by adding olive oil and coriander leaves

**Nutrition:**

Calories: 128

Fat: 8gm

Protein: 4 gm

Carbohydrates: 12 gm

Fibre: 4 gm

## 25. Vegan spinach soup recipe

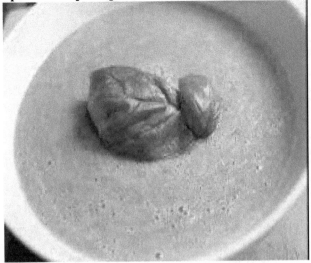

Vegan spinach soup adds another health benefit to your body.

**Time for cooking:** 15-20 minutes

**Cooking ingredients:** 1 medium size onion, 2-3 garlic clove, olive oil 1tablespoon, 400gm fresh spinach leaves, 2 potatoes, vegetable broth, salt and pepper

**Cooking instructions:**
Wash out the spinach leaves, peeled onion, garlic, and potato. Cut all the ingredients into small dices.
Take a pan and heat oil in it. Now add onion, garlic and stir them for few minutes till the raw smell is gone and becomes tender.
Once it is done, add spinach leaves and stir it for 5 to 6 minutes till it softens and wilted.
Now add diced tomatoes and vegetable broth and cook them until tender for 15 to 20 minutes. Once it is done allow the mixture to cool it down and blend it. Pour soup in a bowl add a pinch of salt and black pepper into it.
Garnish it with fresh cream and serve it.

**Nutrition:**
Calorie: 130,
carbohydrate: 24.5 g,
Protein: 4.5 gm,
fibre 5 gm
Fat: 4.1 gm.

## 26. Broccoli rice with cheese

This is a perfect side dish for your fat-filled dinner.

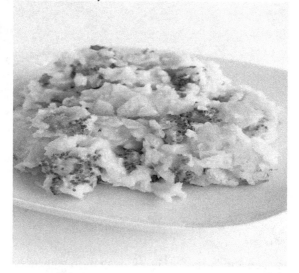

**Cooking time:** 15-20 min

**Ingredients:** 1 cauliflower head riced
1 stalk of broccoli riced
Olive oil 2 tablespoon
1 tablespoon mustard powder
I tablespoon onion powder
1 cup cream
2 cup cheddar cheese
A pinch of salt

**Method to cook:** Heat olive oil in a non-stick pan. Now place garlic, onion and mustard powder into it.
Pour the cream and whisk it gently. Once it did add more cheese into it and stir it occasionally and check the whole cheese has melted.
Add the rice broccoli and cauliflower into the prepared sauce
Boil the mixture till it softens so that excess water is reduced. Stir the mixture continuously to avoid burning of the cheese. Add some salt into it and once the thick cream mixture is formed remove from heat and serve it into the bowl and enjoy it.

**Nutrition:**
Calories: 160
Fat: 15.3 gm
Carbohydrates: 6.2 gm
Proteins: 3 gm

## 27. Broccoli cheese balls

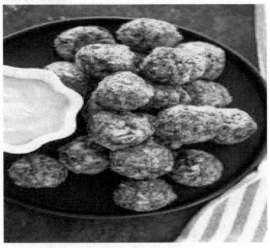

These healthy broccoli bites loaded with cheese, herbs, and spices. This is rich in nutrition and low in carbs and can serve as both a lunch dish and a side dish.

**Total cooking time:** 35 min

**Ingredients:** 3 cups broccoli florets
½ cup almond flour or whole-grain bread crumbs
1 cup mozzarella cheese cubes or shredded
2 eggs
2 tablespoons cilantro optional
1 clove garlic minced
Salt
Black pepper for taste
Seasoning blend or herbs optional

**Cooking method:**
Preheat microwave oven at 350°F. Now lined up baking tray in it
Steam the broccoli by putting them into a microwave bowl and steam it for 2 mins and if steaming in water put some water in the steamer basket and steam until it fully tender
Mix the chopped broccoli, eggs, almond flour cheese, parsley, and spices in a bowl
Make small round balls from the mixture and placed it on the lined baking sheet and spray little oil on it.
Bake it for 25 min or until it goes golden brown
Serve it as you want as lunch, in a sandwich, or a snack with your cheese dips.

**For vegan version-** you can also replace the cheese with vegan cheese and eggs with flax eggs

**Nutrition:** Calorie: 32 per serving
Fat: 2 %
Cholesterol: 12mg
Carbohydrate: 1g
Proteins: 4 gm
Calcium: 3.7%

## 28. Root vegetable lasagna recipe

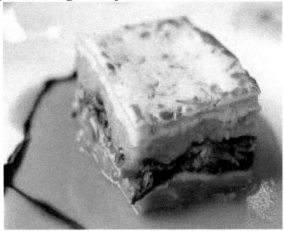

**Cooking time:** 1 hour and 30 minutes

**Cooking ingredients:** 3 and a half cup peeled sweet potato cubed
5 cups peeled butternut squash cubed
2 cups roughly chopped onions
$1/4^{th}$ teaspoon nutmeg grounded
$1/4^{th}$ teaspoon cinnamon powder
2 tablespoon olive oil
2 bay leaves
4 cup milk
2 cups grated Parmigiano-Reggiano cheese
all-purpose flour $1/4^{th}$ cup
Table salt
Black pepper
2 cups shredded mozzarella cheese
Boiled lasagna noodles

**Cooking procedure:**

Preheat oven at 400°F.

Mix the sweet potatoes, chopped onions, and olive oil in a bowl to mix properly. Now place mixture in microwave container and microwave it for 30 minutes

Now in another bowl mix 1 cup onion, cinnamon powder, nutmeg and bay leaf and pour it into pan and bring it to boil. After boiling keep it aside.

Strain the mixture and return the milk into the pan. Now add flour, salt, and pepper to milk mixture. Cook on low flame for 10-12 min. Mix Parmigiano-Reggiano cheese in the mixture.

Now spread this mixture on a baking tray. Arrange the noodles over the mixture, and repeat it to make layers and in last sprinkle some mozzarella cheese. Now, bake it for 30 min.

Now serve it hot as a main dish.

**Nutrition:**

Calories: 254

Protein: 14 gm

Sodium: 300 mg

Sugars: 3gm

## 29. Seasonal fruit salsa with crispy tortillas recipe

Most people missed salsa when they are on the plant paradox diet. But this salsa can be a part of your plant paradox diet which gives your mouth a kick of flavours of fruits.

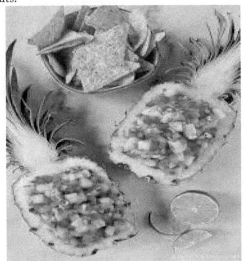

**Cooking time:** 10 to 15 min

**Ingredients:** Apple, berries, peaches, avocado, mango, lime juice, pineapple, poppy seeds, honey

**Cooking method:**
Diced all the fruits,
Add all the ingredients into the bowl and mix them well.
Serve it with crispy tortillas

**Nutrition:**

calories: 94

Fats: 3 percent

Proteins: 4 percent

Vitamins: 50%

## 30. Flaxseed wraps (keto and vegan)

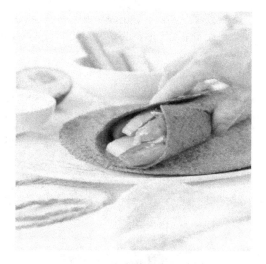

**Total time to cook:** 12 minutes

**Ingredients:** 1 cup flax seeds, 1 teaspoon salt, ¼ teaspoon turmeric, 1 cup water, ¼ teaspoon grated ginger, ¼ teaspoon garlic powder, onion flakes 1 spoon.

**Cooking instructions:** Add flaxseed in a blender and blend them to make a smooth meal.
Now take a saucepan and add water in it and bring it to boil. When water boil, mix it in flaxseed slowly and stir it slowly to make the dough.
Now take a dough ball and place it on parchment paper and make the shape of the tortilla. On medium flame cook these for 1-2 minutes.
Now put wrap in a plate and serve it by adding your favourite toppings as you want.
I use onions flakes to fill in the warp. Serve it and enjoy it.

**Nutrition:**

Calories: 330,

Fat: 26g,

Carbohydrates: 18g,

Sugar: 1g,

Protein: 11g

### 31. Spicy shrimp Taco lettuce wraps

This lettuce wraps makes an amazing dinner or lunch with shrimp and avocado.

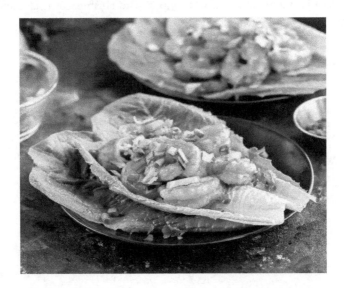

**Total cooking time:** 15 min

**Cooking ingredients:** 1 tablespoon oil (avocado, olive oil)
15 shrimps peeled and divided
1 clove minced garlic
½ teaspoon chili powder
½ teaspoon cumin grounded
Lemon juice
For avocado salsa (1 avocado chunk, 1/3$^{rd}$ cup cilantro leaves chopped, salt, black pepper)
For cilantro sauce (1 clove garlic, ¼ cup sour cream, ¼ cup cilantro, 1 tablespoon lime juice, salt, black pepper,)
10 lettuce leaves

**Cooking instructions:** To make avocado salsa take a bowl and mix all the ingredients and mix thoroughly and keep it aside.

Now bring a bowl put all ingredients like olive oil, garlic, cumin, chili powder, salt and whisk them gently. Add shrimps into the mixture, mix them well so that shrimp coated with the seasoning.

Now take a pan heat oil in it, add olive oil, shrimps in pan and cook for few minutes. Once it is cooked, turn off the heat and keep aside.

Now make the cilantro sauce by adding sour cream, garlic, cilantro, salt, pepper into a food processor and grind them well until creamy texture observed.

Now place two lettuce leaves and topped with shrimps and salsa and serve it with cilantro sauce.

## Nutrition:

Calorie: 230

Fat: 14.2g

Cholesterol: 30mg

Carbohydrate: 22.1g

Fibre: 3.6 g

Protein: 6.7g

Vitamin A and C: 48%

## 32. The roasted vegetables with carb

The low carb roasted vegetables will serve as a simple dish that can easily pair up with any kind of dish. It can be included in both keto diet as well as plant paradox diet.

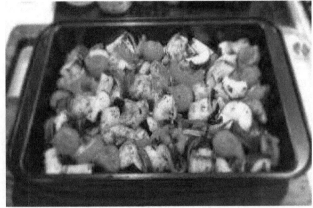

**Cooking time:** 40 min

**Ingredients:** Small head of broccoli
1 zucchini
Half cup olive oil
1 squash
3 bell peppers (red, yellow, green)
10 brussels sprouts
3-4 garlic clove minced
Lime juice
Salt
black pepper
Vinegar
Oregano and parsley

**Cooking Instructions:** Preheat the oven and chop all the vegetables in the same size and placed them into the bowl.

Combine all the above listed ingredients, prepare marinade by adding olive oil, vinegar, salt black pepper. Pour the prepared marinade over vegetables.

Put all veggies on baking sheet by greasing it and bake them for 12 min. But if you are using pan stir them occasionally.

If you want to roast them more then keep it for 5-10 min more.

Once it is done, place them on a plate and pour some lime juice on them and serve them.

**Nutrition:**

Calorie: 131

Carbohydrates: 7gm

Protein: 3 gm

Fat: 11 gm

Fibre: 3 gm

## 33. The green muffins (Gluten-free)

These green muffins are made from fresh spinach, gluten-free oats, honey, and banana. This can be served for breakfast and also be loved by kids.

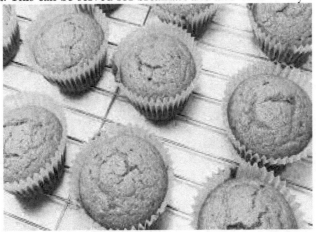

**Cooking time:** 25 min

**Ingredients:** ½ cup water, 1 ripe banana, ¼ cup almond butter, ¼ teaspoon baking soda, 2 spoons honey, 1-2 cups spinach, 1 cup gluten-free oats, ½ teaspoon vanilla extract, ¼ teaspoon ground cinnamon, 1/6th teaspoon salt, 1 egg for vegan version use flax instead of eggs.

**Cooking instructions:**
Preheat the oven at 350°F and grease the muffin tin properly.
Now pour the ingredients into the blender and blend until a smooth paste-like consistency is observed.
Now pour the batter into muffin cups and makes sure grease them well and put these muffins tins into the oven for about 15-17 min till golden brown colour and a bit crack are observed.
Once it is done bring muffins out from oven. Let muffins cool for 30 min and remove them from muffin tin. Store muffins in airtight containers and serve when you want to eat.

**Nutrition: per muffin**
Calories: 47,
fat: 2 gm,
fibre: 0gm,
Protein: 1 gm,
carbohydrates: 6gm.

## 34. Sorghum Salad with dandelion

The healthiest eating with loads of fibre and vitamins and low carb that can serve as a side and main dish both!

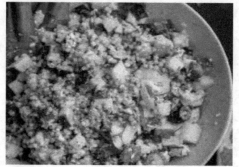

**Total time to cook:** 1 hour and 15 min

**Ingredients:**
2 tablespoon olive oil
2 pounds carrots peeled and cut in an inch size pieces
3 ounces dandelion greens cut into 2-inch pieces
1 bay leaf
5-6 garlic clove
Salt, grounded pepper
1 cup yogurt
3 sprigs thyme
1 cup Sorghum cooked
½ cup celery leaves

**Directions:**
Preheat the oven to 350°F

Now toss all the carrots, garlic, bay leaf with oil and thyme on a baking tray. Add some salt and pepper and let them roast until soft and caramelized for about 35-40 min.
Mash the garlic cloves in bowl, pour yogurt into it and whisk it. Now add some salt and black pepper. Let it stand for 30 minutes. After that spread this yogurt on serving plate and top with sorghum and roasted carrots.
Pour some olive oil and ass some seasonings ns sprinkle some celery leaves and serve it immediately.

**Nutrition:** Calorie: 200
Carbohydrates: 132gm
Protein: 20gm
Fat: 6gm

## 35. Shrimp, avocado and asparagus salad

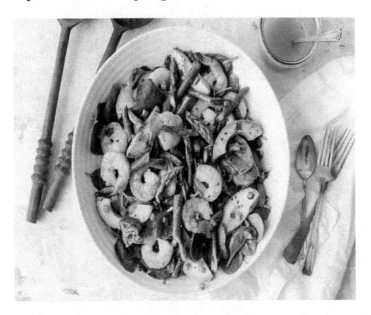

**Total cooking time:** 25 min

**Cooking ingredients:** 1pound shrimp, peeled, 3 cups blanched spinach, 15 asparagus, 1 avocado sliced, spring onion 3 sliced, lemon, salt, and black pepper.

**Method to cook:** Take a pan to add some water and salt in it. Now add shrimp and asparagus and cook them for 2-3 minutes.
When it is done, shift them into the cold water and after that drain them. Cut the asparagus into small pieces.
Now combine all remaining ingredients into bowl toss them. Serve it fresh.

**Nutrition:**
Calorie: 230,
Carbohydrate: 7g,
Protein: 27g,
Fat: 10g,
Cholesterol: 180mg,
Fibre: 4g.

### 36. The green salad with apple cider honey Vinaigrette

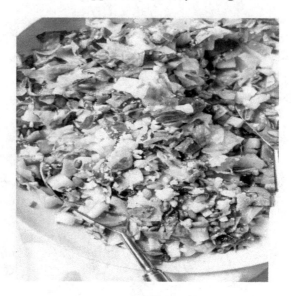

**Total cooking time:** 25 min

**Cooking ingredients:** For salad (3 kiwi fruits peeled and chopped, 4 cups blanched baby spinach, 2 celery ribs, finely sliced. 1 pear sliced ½ cup walnuts, 1 cup goat cheese crushed.

For vinaigrette (1 teaspoon mustard seeds, ½ cup olive oil, honey 1 tablespoon, salt)

**Cooking instructions:**

Whisk all the ingredients of vinaigrette in bowl till they combine.

Now take another bowl combine all salad ingredients and drizzle some amount of vinaigrette on top. Toss to combine and serve them fresh.

**Nutrition:**
Calorie: 90
Fat: 7g
Carbohydrate: 6g
Protein: 0.3g

## 37. The lemon spaghetti with spinach

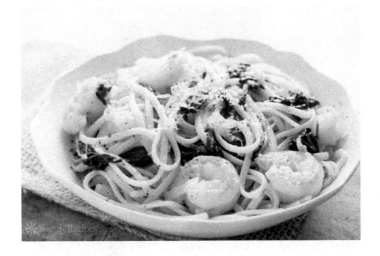

**Total cooking time:** 20 min

**Cooking ingredients:** 1 onion chopped, coconut oil 1 cup, 2 cup vegetable broth, spaghetti 9 oz, 2-3 cup spinach, lemon juice, 2-3 cloves garlic minced, 1 teaspoon lemon zest, red pepper flakes, salt, black pepper.

**Cooking Instructions:** Heat oil in a pan and sauté onion in it for 3 min until they become translucent. After that put garlic in it and cook for another couple of min.

Now put spaghetti, vegetable broth, lemon juice, and coconut milk in the pan. Strengthen it for a couple of minutes and let them cook for 10 minutes.

Once the spaghetti is done stir the spinach and add lemon zest and cook for 2 minutes.
Serve it by adding seasonings like salt, pepper, chili flakes.

**Nutrition:**
Calorie: 400,
Carbohydrates: 60,
Protein: 12g,
Fat: 14g,
Fibre: 7g,
Vitamin A 50%.

## 38. Apple walnut spinach salad with vinaigrette

This delicious winter salad packed with healthy nutrition.

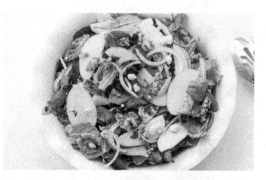

**Total time to cook:** 30 min

**Ingredients:**
For salad
1 apple sliced
5 cup spinach
1 cup chopped walnuts
½ small onion sliced
½ cup goat cheese
½ cup blue cheese

For dressing
2 tablespoon maple syrup
2 tablespoon olive oil
3 tablespoon balsamic vinegar
½ teaspoon Dijon mustard

**Cooking instructions:** Take a bowl and put all the ingredients into it. Mix all ingredients properly.

Now whisk the dressing ingredients into a bowl and pour this on the salad. Toss them well so that the mixture gets fully incorporated and top them with goat cheese and blue cheese.

**Nutrition:**
Calorie: 260,
Carbohydrate: 32g,
Fibre: 3g,
Protein: 7g,
Vitamin A: 90%

### 39. The cauliflower crust spinach pizza

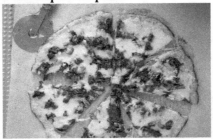

**Cooking time:** 40 min
**Serving:** 8

**Ingredients:** 1 medium head cauliflower, crushed and finely chopped
½ teaspoon black pepper for the crust
1 egg
½ cup low-fat cheese
½ cup oregano
½ teaspoon of sea salt
2 and half cup spinach
Fresh or sun-dried tomatoes
One cup mozzarella cheese

**Cooking instructions:**

Preheat oven at 300 degrees. Now place baking tray in it grease it with olive oil.

Now transfer the finely chopped cauliflower into the microwave dish and microwave it for about 8 minutes till it cooked. Please make sure that there is no water that remains in the cauliflower as it will end up in the mushy dough

Now transfer the cauliflower in a bowl and add an egg into it. Now add some mozzarella cheese, oregano, salt, and black pepper and then press this mixture on the baking tray to make pizza base and cook it till it becomes golden brown for 15 min.

Side by side, cook spinach in a pan till it gets wilted.
Scatter it on the base, add mozzarella cheese and sun-dried tomatoes, and salt.
Bake it for another 10 min till the cheese melts.
Serve it hot.

**Nutrition:** Calorie: 169, Carbohydrate: 5.8 gm
Fat: 2.1 gm, Fibre: 1.2gm, Protein: 5.1 gm

# 40. The pumpkin soup

The pumpkin soup is keto-friendly, low carb, and a healthy appetizer that serves as a main dish.

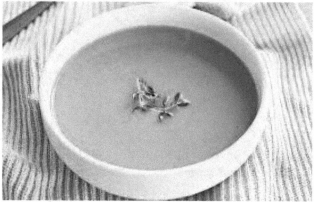

**Cooking time:** 20 min

**Ingredients:** Pumpkin puree, 2 cups vegetable broth, ½ tablespoon pepper and salt, 1 teaspoon garlic powder, ½ cup fresh cream, chopped parsley, roasted pumpkin seeds

**Cooking method:**

Pour the puree of pumpkin and vegetable broth in a pan and also add garlic, thyme and stir it to mix them all.
Bring it to boil, now reduce flame and cook for another 10 minutes. Once it done remove from flame. Pour this into the serving bowl and garnish with fresh cream, roasted seeds, and parsley.

**Nutrition:** Amount per serving
Calories: 120
Fat; 30%
Cholesterol: 32mg
Carbohydrates: 7gm
Protein: 2gm

## 41. The anti-inflammatory egg soups

This anti-inflammatory egg soup takes less than 20 minutes to prepare. This soup is best suits to boost your immune system and loads you with antioxidants and anti-inflammatory action.

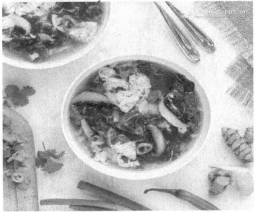

**Cooking time:** 20 min

**Ingredients:** 2 cups vegetable broth, 1 tablespoon turmeric freshly grated, 2 cloves minced garlic, 1 tablespoon ginger freshly grated, 2 cup brown mushroom sliced, chard leaves, 1 cup Chile pepper, 3 cup chopped spinach, 3 medium spring onions, 4 eggs, 2 tablespoon freshly chopped cilantro, olive oil, salt to taste.

**Cooking instructions:**
Take a pan pour vegetable broth in it and bring it to a boil. Now place grated ginger, turmeric, garlic, sliced mushroom, Chile pepper into the broth and bring to boil for 5 min.

After this add chard leaves and slowly add eggs into the simmering soup. Now pour this soup into a serving bowl and add some olive oil into it and serve it

**Nutrition:**
calories: 255,
Fat: 22.4 gm,
Protein: 10.8 gm
carbohydrates: 2 gm,
fat: 50gm.

## 42. Vegetarian ramen (low carbs)

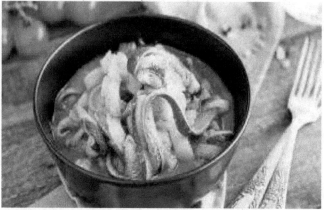

**Cooking time:** 30 minutes

**Cooking ingredients:** purple cabbage chopped 1 cup, shredded carrots 1 cup, 1 cups brussels sprouts, 1 large zucchini, 4 eggs, 2 cup coconut milk, coconut oil, chili flakes, cilantro 1 tablespoon ginger grated, garlic, turmeric, 1 lime juice, salt, pepper, 4 cups water. 1 cup curry paste with chili-infused.

**Cooking instructions:**
In a pot, pour water and bring it to boil. When water boils prepare some chili infusion. Take a pan heat oil in it, add chili flakes, sizzle it for 5 min and keep it aside.

In the boiling water add coconut milk and spices. Now add cabbage, carrots, Brussels and curry paste into it and cook for another 20 min. Boil some egg in another pan for 6 minutes.

When the vegetables are done, add zucchini and cook for 3-4 minutes
Now serve the vegetable ramen with eggs, lime juice, and cilantro and chili-infused oil.

**Nutrition:**
calories: 230,
Fat: 12gm,
Cholesterol: 180mg,
Fibre: 4 gm,
protein: 10gm

### 43. Low carb Cheesy pepperoni wheel pizza

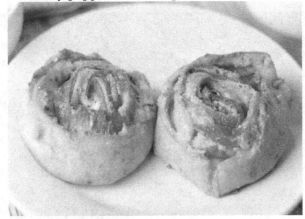

**Total cooking time:** 25 min

**Ingredients:** For making the dough (1 teaspoon onion powder, 3 tablespoon coconut flour, 1 teaspoon garlic powder, Italian seasonings 1 teaspoon, ¼ cup almond flour, ½ teaspoon salt and black pepper, 1 cup mozzarella cheese shredded, Butter 1 tablespoon, 2 tablespoon cream cheese, 1 egg)
for filling (1 cup mozzarella cheese, ½ cup pizza sauce, ½ cup parmesan cheese, 4 pepperoni slices, Italian seasonings)

**Cooking method:** Preheat microwave oven at 375°F.
Now take bowl put all ingredients like flours, garlic powder, onion powder, salt, seasonings, black pepper and mix them well to make dough.
 In another bowl combine all the cheese and microwave them for a minute to melt it. now add eggs and all other ingredients and microwave them for 20-30 seconds.
Once it is done spread the dough on parchment paper and make a thin layer from it. Now spread the pizza sauce and put another layer of mozzarella cheese and top them with pepperoni slices. Sprinkle some seasoning over the top.
Now roll the dough into slices and make wheels from them. Bake these rolls for 15 minutes till they got fluffy and golden brown. Once it is done serve them hot.

**Nutrition:**
Calorie: 230,
Fat: 16g,
Protein: 12g,
carbs: 7g,
Fibre: 3g

# 44. The millets noodles recipe

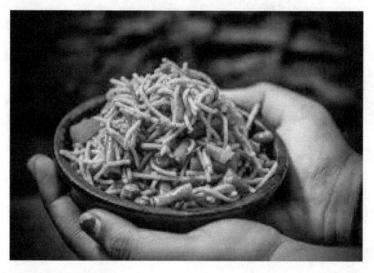

**Cooking time:** 15-20 min

**Ingredients:** 1 pack millet noodles, 1 tablespoon olive oil, Garlic 2,3 cloves thin sliced. 2 medium onions, chilli 2, cabbage ½ cup, carrots ½ cups, 1 tablespoon soy sauce, green chili sauce 1 tablespoon, tomato sauce 1 spoon, salt, black pepper ¼ teaspoon, spring onions ½ cup.

**Cooking Instructions:** Take a pan put water, noodles and boil the noodles for 5 min until they become soft. Now pour the noodles in the sieve, rinse with chilled water and keep it aside for drain.

Now take other pan and heat oil in it, put some garlic and Sauté for 2 minutes and slowly put onions, green chilies in it. When it's done add cabbage and carrot and let them fry for 2-3 minutes.

Now add soy sauce, green chili sauce, and salt and mix them well.

Remove the cooked noodles from the flame and garnish with coriander leaves. serve them hot with tomato sauce as a main dish.

**Nutrition:**
Calorie: 130
Fat: 1.5 gm
cholesterol: 0mg
Carbohydrates: 24gm
Protein: 4 gm

## 45. Millet mushroom risotto

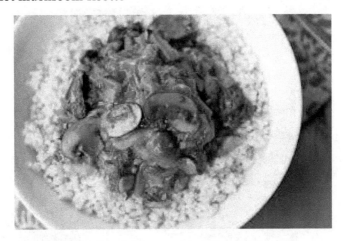

**Cooking time:** soaking time 2-3 hours or whole night
Preparing time: 20 min

### Ingredients:

1 cup millet, soaked overnight
1 clove garlic crushed
mushroom, thin sliced 1 cup
1 onion chopped
1 cup swiss button mushroom, sliced
2 tablespoon sesame oil or olive oil
2 tablespoon white miso paste
3 cups vegetable broth
Salt to taste
Parsley

**Cooking Instructions:** In a pan, add millet and vegetables both, and bring it to boil till it absorbs the broth and becomes fluffy.

Take a pan heat sesame oil in it and toss garlic, onion until they get soft and translucent. Now add Mushrooms toss it till soften. Now add millet and miso paste and stir it for a min and add salt. Remove from flame
Serve it on a plate by sprinkling parsley.

### Nutrition:
Calorie: 230
Fat: 13.6 gm
Cholesterol: 17.0 mg
Carbohydrate: 18.3 gm
Fibre: 1.5gm

### 46. Vegan curry ramen

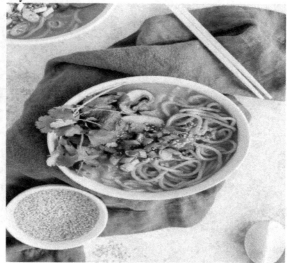

**Total cooking time:** 20 minutes

**Ingredients:** 1 cup shredded carrots, 8 sliced mushroom, 2 tablespoon red curry paste, 1 cup sugar peas, 1 tablespoon sesame oil, 7 cloves minced garlic, minced ginger 2 tablespoon, coconut milk 1 cup, 5 cup vegetable broth, curry powder 2 tablespoon, 1 tablespoon lime juice, ramen noodles, salt, pepper, chopped cilantro, jalapeno, lime slices.

**Cooking instructions:**

Heat sesame oil in pan add carrots, mushrooms, peas and toss them for few minutes. Add salt and pepper in it and mix them thoroughly.

Once it has done add curry paste, garlic, ginger, and curry powder, cook it for couple of minutes. Now add coconut milk and vegetable broth in it. Now add salt and black pepper in it as per your taste and keep this aside.
Now add ramen noodles into it and cook for another 10 minutes. Squeeze lemon juice on it, garnish with cilantro, jalapeno and lemon slices.

**Nutrition:**
Calorie: 285,
Fat: 16g,
Cholesterol: 0.0mg,
Carbohydrates: 32g,
Fibre: 4g,
Sugar: 5g.

## 47. Kohlrabi celeriac soup (the clean eating soup)

When you want to reduce some extra pounds and want some low carb food then this soup will serve you the best. The kohlrabi helps in eliminating excess toxins from the body thus act as a cleanser. Take a look at how you can prepare for this.

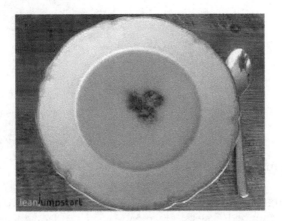

**Cooking time:** 30 min

**Ingredients:** kohlrabi 300g, peeled and cut in small cubes, 300g celeriac bulb, peeled, cut in small cubes, 1 tablespoon olive oil, 500ml vegetable broth, 1 leek chopped, 200 ml coconut milk, nutmeg, salt, pepper, parsley

**Cooking instructions:** Take a saucepan and heat oil in that.

Now add kohlrabi cubes, celeriac cubes, and leek and sauté them for 2 min
Now add vegetable broth in it and bring it to boil. Let it boil on low flame for 20 min.
Now add coconut milk and make puree till smooth. Add some more broth for perfect consistency.
Add salt, pepper, and nutmeg and place it in a bowl and garnish with parsley and serve hot

**Nutrition:**

Calorie: 36 per serving

Vitamin B6 and C: 50%

Carbs: 8gm

Protein: 13g

Fat: 0.3 g

## 48. Creamy Avocado-leek soup

This soup can be served in dinner and as an appetizer.

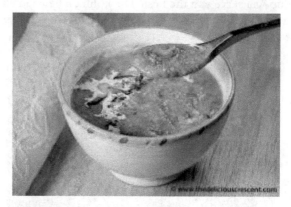

**Cooking time: 30 minutes**

**Cooking ingredients:** olive oil 1 tablespoon, 1 onion peeled and chopped, 1 garlic clove chopped, 2 leeks (green part only chopped), 400g white beans, 400ml vegetable broth or chicken broth as suits you, 2 tablespoon apple cider vinegar, 1 avocado skin removed, freshly chopped green onions, salt, black pepper.

**Cooking Instructions:** Take a pan heat oil in it, add some leeks into oil and fry for 3-4 min until it got light brown coloured. Now remove the leek from the flame.

Put some onion and garlic into the pan and stir them till they become translucent. Now add vegetable broth, vinegar, and beans and boil it for 15 min by covering the lid.

Once it did let the soup cool down before blending. Now add avocado, salt, pepper and blend the soup until it forms a smooth consistency and returns into the pan. Reheat the soup and add more broth or water if needed. Serve the soup topping with green onions.

**Nutrition:**
Calorie: 200
Fat: 5.3 g
Cholesterol: 14.2mg
Carbohydrates: 37 g
Protein: 4.8g

## 49. Roasted Garlic and cauliflower soup

The vegan roasted garlic and cauliflower soup add another healthy option. The antioxidants present in garlic serve you with various health benefits. It can be served at lunch and dinner.

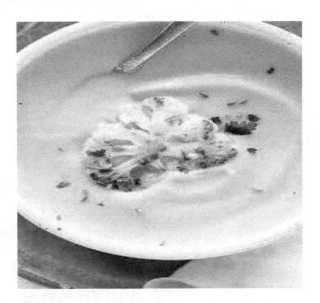

**Cooking time:** 1 hour

**Ingredients:** 2 head cauliflower (cut into small florets).

1 medium-size white onion, diced

2 tablespoon olive oil

2 cups almond milk

4 cups vegetable broth or water

2 garlic cloves peeled and crushed

apple cider vinegar 1 tablespoon

Salt as per taste

black pepper

**Cooking instructions:**

Preheat oven at 400°F. Now link baking tray by parchment paper. Now spread cauliflower florets and garlic cloves on the tray.

Roast the cauliflower and garlic for 30-40 min. Roast these until they got golden brown.

Now bring a pan heat olive oil in it, add onions into oil and toss for 5 to 6 min once the onions get translucent.

Now add roasted cauliflower and garlic into the pan with vegetable broth.

Bring mixture to a boil after that reduces the flame and cook for another 15 min.

Now pour soup into the blender. Blend soup until it gets smooth consistency.

Now pour almond milk, vinegar, salt, pepper in it and blend again.

Pour soup into the bowl. Drizzle some olive oil on it.

**Nutrition:**
Calorie: 300
Fat: 24.2 g
Cholesterol: 40mg
Carbohydrate: 23g
Fibre: 5.6 g
Protein: 13.9 g

## 50. Creamy carrot and ginger soup

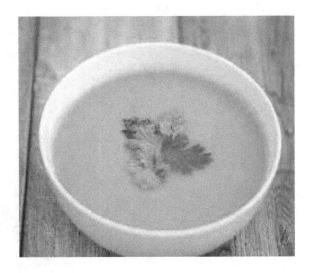

**Cooking time:** 35 min

**Ingredients:** 1 clove garlic, 4 tablespoon ginger chopped, 300 gm carrots peeled and chopped, vegetable broth 2 cup, coconut oil 1 tablespoon, 1 onion chopped, 1 cup coconut milk, salt a pinch and pepper.

**Instructions:** Heat coconut oil in pan on low flame. Now put onion, ginger, garlic into the oil and cook for few minutes or until the raw smell is done.

Now add carrots, vegetable broth into pan and boil it for few minutes. After boil reduce the flame and boil it for another 25 min until the carrots are soft. Now slowly add coconut milk. Once it is done, pour the mixture into the blender and blend the soup until it becomes smooth cream-like consistency. Now add a pinch of salt and pepper as per your taste. Serve hot in a bowl.

**Nutrition:**

Calorie: 280

Fat: 23g

Carbohydrate: 17 g

Fibre: 5 g

Vitamin A and C: 50%

# 51. The clear Japanese soup

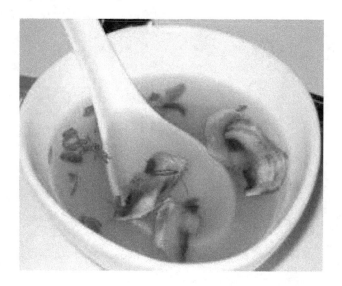

**Cooking time:** 1 hour

**Ingredients:** 2 teaspoon peanut oil, 6 cups chicken broth ( vegetable broth for vegan version), 4 cups water, 1 onion peeled and chopped into small pieces, 3-4 cloves of garlic, peeled and crushed, 2 carrots, cut into small pieces, 2 inch fresh sliced ginger, 4 scallion hopped, 10 buttons of mushroom sliced, salt as per taste.

**Cooking instructions:** Place the stockpot on medium heat and add oil in it. Now add onion, garlic, carrots, and ginger in the oil and stir the veggies till they get softer.

Now pour the broth and water into pot and boil the mixture. After boiling, lower down the flame, cook mixture for one hour. Once it did remove from the flame and pour it into the bowl. Garnish it with chopped scallion, sliced mushrooms, and salt.

**Nutrition: as per cup**
Calorie: 46,
Carbohydrate: 5g,
Protein: 3g,
Fat: 1g
Cholesterol: 0 mg,
Calcium: 35mg.

## 52. Avocado seaweed wraps with cilantro dipping sauce

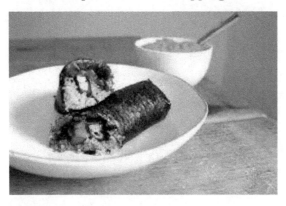

**Time of cooking:** 30 minutes

**Cooking ingredients:** avocado oil 1 tablespoon, 4 ounces breast chicken, 2 tablespoons freshly squeezed lemon juice, ½ avocado diced, 1 cup arugula, sushi seaweed, 4 green olives, pitted and halved.

**For vegan version:** instead of chicken you can use cauliflower streak or hemp tofu

### Cilantro dipping sauce
2 cup chopped cilantro
2 tablespoon lemon juice
extra-virgin olive oil ½ cup
salt ¼ teaspoon

### Cooking instructions:

### For filling

Heat the avocado oil in a pan and place chicken strips in it and fry by adding 1 tablespoon lemon juice and salt and sauté it for about 2-3 min. Once the side is done, flip the side and cook for another 2-3 min.

Now remove the chicken strips from the pan and tossed some avocado in the pan and add lemon juice and salt.

### Dipping sauce

Put cilantro, olive oil, lemon juice, and salt into blender. Blend this mixture until it turns into smooth paste.

For serving:

Arrange arugula on bottom of seaweed sheet

Top this sea weed sheet with chicken, avocado, olives and sprinkle salt on it and role in the form of a wrap.

**Nutrition:**

Calories: 250

Fat: 10gm

Protein: 8gm

Cholesterol: 3mg

Carbohydrates: 20.6 gm

## 53. Cooked lentils chili

The red smokie lentil chili recipe loaded with flavour, protein, and fibre. It is a plant-based meal perfect for lunch and dinner served.

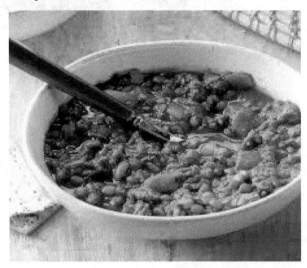

**Cooking time:** 55 min
**Ingredients:**

2 tablespoon avocado oil or coconut oil, 2 red pepper cubed, 2 onions diced, ½ teaspoon salt, black pepper, 1 small jalapeno diced, 4-5 garlic cloves, chilli powder 3 teaspoon, cumin powder 2 teaspoon, paprika 1 tablespoon, 2 diced tomatoes, 3 tablespoon tomato paste, 1 ¾ cup water, ¾ dry red lentils, 1.5 ounces kidney beans, 1-2 teaspoon corn sugar, 1.5 ounces black beans, 1 can dried corn.

**Cooking Instructions:** Take a pan heat oil in it. Now add onions, red pepper and season with salt and stir it for 3-4 min.

Now add jalapenos and crushed garlic and add into the pot with onion and red pepper and add some salt. Now add chili powder, cumin, paprika, tomatoes, and tomato paste and water and boil it on medium flame.

Now add the lentils and cook them on low flame. Cook for 15 min till lentils become soft and tender.

Add some kidney beans, black beans, salt, pepper, cumin powder, and chili powder. and boil for another 15 min to cook.

Once it did serve it hot and add seasonings if needed.

**Nutrition:** Calorie: 117.1, Vitamin: 5 %, Fat: 0.5 gm, protein: 7.6gm, cholesterol: 0.0 mg, sodium: 700mg, potassium: 490mg

## 54. The pasta lectin free

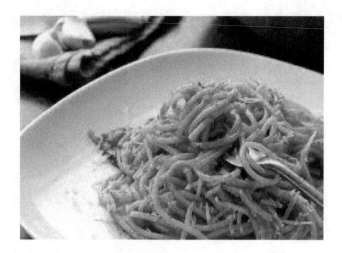

**Total time to cook:** 20 min

**Ingredients:** 1 cup almond flour, tapioca flour1 cup, salt 1 teaspoon, 2 eggs, olive oil.

**Instructions:** Combine tapioca flour, almond flour, salt, and eggs and knead a smooth dough. Once the dough is ready, divide it into small portions.

Roll the dough on board and make a thick layer approximate 1/6 inch thick. Now by using pizza cutter cut noodles of desired length and thickness.

Take a large pan and add water to it. Put a few drops of olive oil in it. Once the water is boiled add noodles into it and bring it to boil till soft for 2 min

Once the noodles are done remove it from the flame, strain it and add some freshwater drain it and drizzle some olive oil on it.

Serve the noodles with curry or soup.

**Nutrition:**
Calorie: 176,
Fat: 1gm,
Cholesterol: 0mg,
Carbohydrate: 30gm,
Protein: 3.8gm

## 55. Almond flour tortillas keto gluten-free recipe

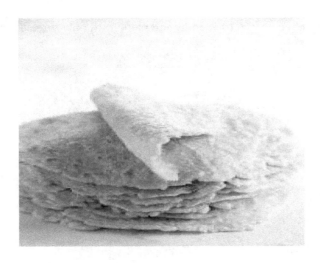

**Total time to cook:** 20 min

**Ingredients:** almond flour 2 cups, baking powder 1 teaspoon, 3 egg whites, water, oil, 1 teaspoon salt, 4 teaspoon psyllium powder.

**Instruction:** Put all the above listed ingredients in a bowl and combine them properly. Now add water to make the dough. Let the dough sit for 5 min. Now make small round balls of the dough and roll it to form thin tortillas. Once these are ready, Heat oil in the pan and place one tortilla inside it and cook from each side for 30 seconds till the crust becomes golden brown.

Repeat the steps with other tortillas.

**Nutrition:** per tortilla

Calorie: 135

Fat: 9.2 g

Cholesterol: 0mg

Carbohydrate: 10.1g

Protein: 5.8g

### 56. Crispy Roasted Red cabbage

This simple recipe is keto-friendly and made with only three basic ingredients.

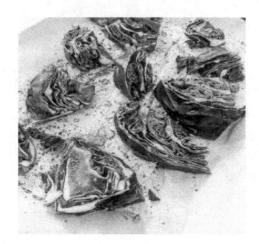

**Total cooking time:** 45 min

**Ingredients:** 1 head red cabbage

Olive oil

2 teaspoon zaatar spice

**Instructions for cooking:** preheat the oven on 375°F

Wash the cabbage and cut it into fine wedges with a knife.

Drizzle olive oil on cabbage and parchment sheet and sprinkle some zaatar seasoning on it

Roast it for about 20 min and slightly toss them and again roast them for 20 min till it becomes crispy. However, timing will depend on the size of the cabbage you have cut.

Once it did serve it to eat.

**Nutrition:**
Calorie: 117,
Fat: 7g,
Cholesterol: 0mg,
carbohydrates: 13g,
fibre: 6g,
Protein: 4g

## 57. Vegan Mushroom Bourguignon with potato cauliflower mash

The vegan gluten-free recipe will add another flavour to your tongue.

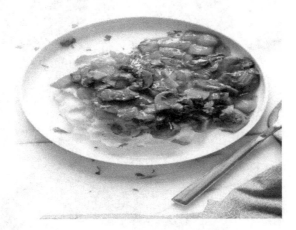

**Cooking time:** 30 min

**Ingredients:** 3-4 cloves of garlic chopped, 2 tablespoon oil, 1 onion chopped, ¾ cup chopped carrots, 2 cups chopped celery, garlic powder ½ teaspoon, soy sauce 1 tablespoon, vegetable broth 1 cup, mushroom 10 buttons sliced, ¼ cup red wine, 1 tablespoon cornstarch,1 cup of spinach.

For potato mash: 1 potato cubes, 1 cup cauliflower florets, olive oil, 1 teaspoon garlic powder, black pepper to taste and coconut milk 1 cup.

**Cooking instruction:** Heat the pot and add oil in it. Now add onion, garlic, mushrooms, and salt and sauté them for 3-4 minutes until they got golden brown.

Now pour some wine in it, mix well. Now put carrots, celery and garlic powder and mix them well. Put soya sauce, salt, and water broth. Now place the steamer basket on top of the mushroom mixture and add potatoes and cauliflower in it.

Close the lid and cook for 9-10 min. Let the pressure release and open the lid. Now transfer the steamed potato and cauliflower into a bowl and mash them. Add some more garlic powder, salt, pepper, olive oil, coconut milk, and fresh herbs.

Serve the mash with mushroom bourguignon. Garnish with basil.

**Nutrition:**

Calorie: 200
Carbohydrate: 8g
Fat: 3.2 g
Cholesterol: 2mg
Protein: 8g

## 58. Creamy mushroom stroganoff
**Cooking time:** 30 min

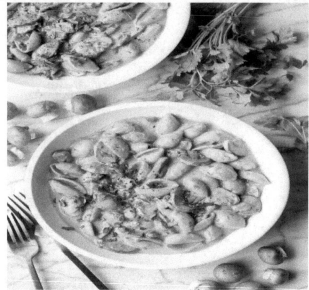

**Ingredients:** pasta shells 2 cup, 2 cup mushrooms sliced, 2 large shallots diced, 3-4 cloves minced garlic, 3 tablespoon butter, 4 teaspoon fresh thyme, all-purpose flour 2 tablespoon, vegetable stock 2 cup, 1 teaspoon mustard seeds, ½ cup sour cream, ½ cup grated parmesan cheese, parsley leaves, salt.

**Cooking Directions:** Pour water in a pan and boil it. Now put pasta in boiling water to boil it.

Take another skillet and heat the butter in it. Now put mushrooms, shallots in skillet, cook for few minutes. Now add a pinch of salt. Now stir it in garlic and thyme for about 1 min and whisk the flour in it till light brown. Now pour the stock in it and bring it to boil.

After boiling reduces flame and cook till it thickened

Now add pasta and sour cream and mix them for 1-2 min. add some parmesan cheese till melt.

Serve in a bowl and garnish them with parsley.

**Nutrition:**
Calorie: 330.6
Fat: 8.9g
Cholesterol: 0.0 mg
Protein: 16g
Carbohydrate: 50g
Fibre: 6.8 g

## 59. Low carb hot dog buns with vegan toppings

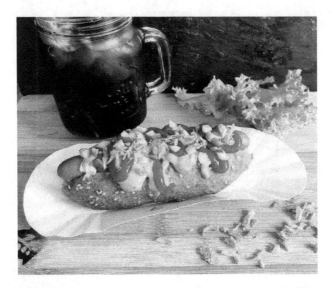

**Cooking time:** 20 min

**Cooking ingredients:** For buns (3 eggs, almond flour 2 cups, baking powder 1 teaspoon)
For toppings (1 onion chopped, olive oil, tossed mushroom 2 buttons, parsley chopped, boiled corn kernels 2 spoons, salt, pepper)

**Cooking Instructions:** Combine the ingredients of bun in bowl. Pour into baking tray and bake it for 2 minutes.
Now cut the bread into equal lengths and keep them into the plate.
Now mix all the toppings and place them into the hot dog buns.
You can also add mustard sauce, mayo sauce as per your taste.

**Nutrition:**
Calories: 300
Fat: 37g
Protein: 12g
Fibre: 3g
Sugar: 2g

## 60. Plantain pancakes

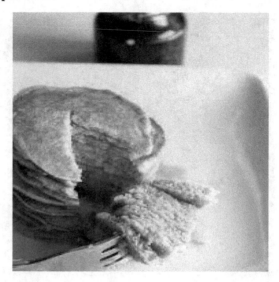

**Cooking time:** 35 min

**Ingredients:** 2 medium-size ripe plantains puree, melted butter 1/3 cup, milk 2/3 cup, flour 1 cup, ¾ cup water, 5 eggs, ¼ cup sugar, 1 teaspoon nutmeg, vanilla extract 1 teaspoon, oil ½ cup if needed

**Method:** Mix all the ingredients until it is fully incorporated and let the batter rest for about 30 min. Now heat the pan and some vegetable oil or butter in it, Spread the batter in the pan and let it cook till it softened and fluffy for about 2-3 minutes.

Once it is done swerve it with coconut sauce and sugar syrup on it.

**Nutrition:**

calories: 398

Fat: 22gm

Cholesterol: 249gm

Carbohydrates: 43mg

Fibre: 2gm

Protein: 9gm

## 61. Sweet Potato gluten-free crusted quiche with leeks and cheese

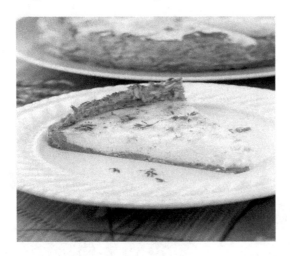

**Cooking time:** 50 min

**Cooking ingredients:**
For crust (1 tablespoon salt, 2 sweet potatoes peeled grated, 1 teaspoon pepper, red pepper flakes, 1 egg)
For the filling (1 leek white and green part sliced, 2 tablespoon butter, 6 eggs, ½ teaspoon salt, ½ teaspoon pepper, ½ cup coconut milk, 3 cup goat cheese crushed)

**Cooking Instructions:** Preheat the oven at 400°F and grease the bottom of the baking pan with cooking oil.
Now take parchment paper and cut into circles. Line up sheet and grease it with cooking spray.
Now place the grated sweet potato in a muslin cloth to squeeze the extra water.
Now take a bowl and whisk egg, salt, red pepper flakes, black pepper and mix grates sweet potato into it. Now on bottom of pan press sweet potato mixture and bake it for 30 min.

Now heat the butter and add leeks in it. Sprinkle a pinch of pepper, salt and cook for 8 min.
Prepare egg mixture by adding coconut milk, cream, salt, and pepper to make a smooth paste. Add the mixture into the sweet potato pan by adding goat cheese in it and bake it for 30 min. Once it is done serve it hot.

**Nutrition:** Calorie: 240, Fat: 16g, Cholesterol: 160mg, carbohydrate: 11g, protein: 12g.

## 62. Shrimp Scampi Pasta

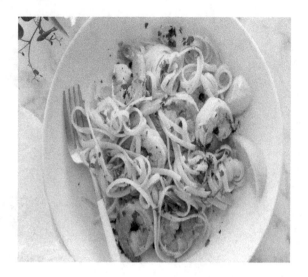

**Cooking time:** 30 min

**Cooking Ingredients:** 15 shrimps peeled and thawed
2 tablespoon olive oil
2 tablespoon butter
¼ cup lemon juice
One hand full chopped parsley
Salt
Pepper
1 lemon cut into small wedges
1 pinch red chili flakes
1 cup pasta

**Cooking Instructions:** Melt butter in the pan and add olive oil, shrimp and sauté it for 3-5 min.
Add garlic and boiled pasta, lemon wedges, red chili flakes and toss them for 3-4 minutes
Serve it immediately or hot.

**Nutrition:**
Calorie: 400,
Fat: 29g,
Cholesterol: 20mg,
Protein: 26.5 g,
Carbohydrate: 4.9g

## 63. Sweet potato hash

It is a healthy vegetarian side dish that is easy to cook and can be taken as a full meal.

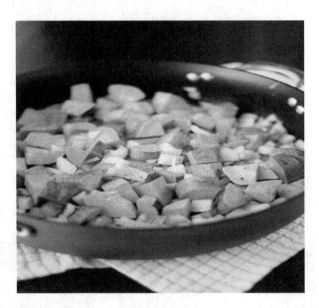

**Time for cooking:** 30 minutes

**Cooking ingredients:** 3 sweet potatoes sliced, 2 stalks celery chopped, 2 tablespoon olive oil, 1 onion diced, salt, 2 cloves garlic minced, sliced green onion.

**Cooking Instructions:** Take a pan heat oil in it, put sweet potatoes, onion, celery in it and stir to mix them properly. Sprinkle some salt when it is done and pepper for taste. Now cover the lid of the pan for 20 min and cook it. Occasionally stir it to avoid burning. Now add garlic and cook it for another 5 min. Cook it until sweet potato gets soften.
Serve it hot and garnish it with spring onion

**Nutrition:**
Calories: 170,
Fat: 6g, Protein: 6g,
Fibre: 4.2g,
Sugar: 6g,
Cholesterol: 0.0mg

## 64. Tabbouleh with millet and hemp
**Total cooking time:** 30 min

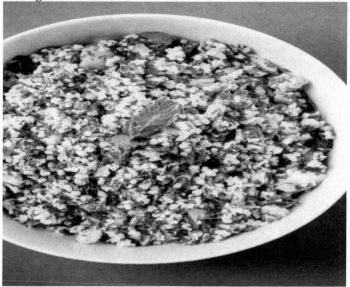

**Cooking ingredients:** 3 tablespoon hemp, red reddish 6 finely chopped, one bunch of parsley finely chopped, 4 tablespoon olive oil, 3 spring onions (finely chopped), 2/4th cup cooked millet, 1 lemon zest, ¼ cup finely chopped olives, lemon juice 1 spoon, salt, pepper for taste.

**Cooking instructions:** for cooking millets roast them into the pan and add water mix it and add some salt and let it boil for 15 min. Now remove this from heat.
Take another pan and add oil and mix all the finely chopped veggies and herbs into it. Sauté them for few minutes and add cooked millets and hemp with lemon zest and olive oil. Mix all the ingredients and add lemon juice into it. You can serve it or refrigerate it for further use.

**Nutrition:** per serving

Calories: 82

Fat: 4.1g

Fibre: 3.4g

Sugar: 3.5g

Protein: 4g

## 65. Spring vegetables with fettuccine alfredo

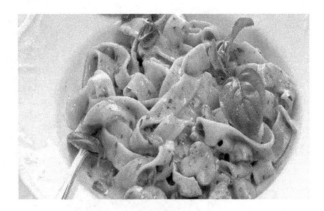

**Total cooking time:** 30 minutes

**Cooking ingredients:** ½ cup extra-virgin olive oil, whole grain pasta, 2 cups sliced mushrooms, ½ bunch asparagus cuts into pieces, 1 lemon zest, 1 cup Italian mascarpone, ½ cup Parmigiano-Reggiano grated, ½ cup chopped parsley leaves, black pepper, 1 teaspoon seasoning, salt.

**Cooking instructions:**

Take a pan pour water and pasta in it and boil it till it cooked. Now drain the water and toss the pasta in oil.

Now take a pan heat oil in it and toss mushroom into it on high flame. Stir it for 2-3 minutes. Once it is done add some more olive oil and toss asparagus into it. Now add a pinch of salt and cook them for two minutes.

Now turn off flame, add the remaining ingredients and pasta into it. Toss them so that it is cooked full and salt and pepper. Add the remaining water of pasta. Garnish it with seasoning and serve them hot.

**Nutrition:** calories: 234, Fat: 6g, Protein: 9g, carbohydrates: 6g, Fibre: 7g

### Healthy snacks items

When we think about snacks a sudden thing strikes to mind is a lot of cheese, spices, fried food and lot more carbohydrates and sugars. So, when we are following any keto diet, plant paradox diet, the first thing that comes to our mind is we have to quit snacks by killing our wish to eat them. But here you don't need to worry we have keeping your heart a bit above by including healthy keto snacks with low carbohydrates and keto-friendly that will indirectly supply nutrients to your body. Let's take a look at these delicious snack recipes.

## 66. Zucchini chips

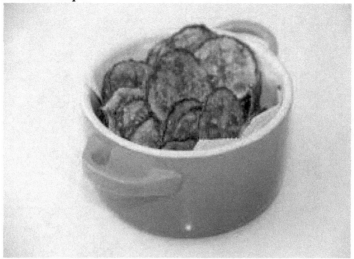

**Cooking time:** 1 hour 40 min

**Ingredients:** Cooking spray, 2 zucchinis finely sliced
olive oil 1 tablespoon
dried oregano 1 teaspoon
Salt
pepper

**Directions:** Preheat the oven at 225°F. Now grease baking tray with cooking oil or spray. Now put sliced zucchini on the baking tray, pat dry with paper towels to remove excess water. Bake until it got crispy for about 1 hour and store them in airtight containers. Add seasoning and oregano and salt on the chips.

If you are using air fryer then you air fry at 375° for about 6-7 mins.

## 67. Keto cinnamon rolls

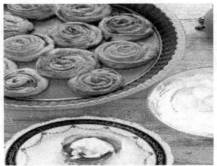

**Cooking time:** 1 hour 20 min
**Ingredients:**
For rolls
Almond flour 2 cups
2 tablespoon coconut flour
¼ cups stevia
2 eggs
baking powder 1 teaspoon
vanilla extract 2 teaspoon
2 cup shredded mozzarella
3 tablespoons butter
cream cheese 4 ounces
ground cinnamon 1 teaspoon
2 tablespoon heavy cream
**Directions:** Take a bowl put all ingredients including coconut flour, almond flour, baking powder and mix them until incorporated fully. Take another bowl, whisk vanilla extract and eggs.
In another microwave bowl, microwave mozzarella and cream cheese for about 90 sec. Now add egg mixture and melted cheese mixture and knead until combined.
Now turn the dough on parchment paper and turn the dough on paper and place another piece of parchment on top and rolls until takes the shape of a rectangular sheet. brush them with melted butter, brown sugar and cinnamon and bake it for 30 min till golden brown.
Serve with drizzle icing over rolls.

**Nutrition:**
Calorie: 383,
Carbs: 37gm,
Fat: 8gm,
Protein: 8gm

### 68. Cassava flour waffles

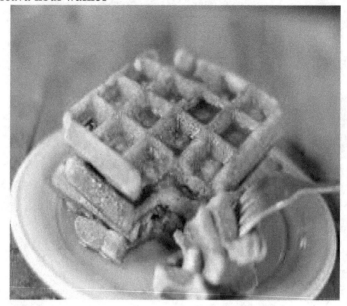

**Cooking time:** 25 min

**Ingredients:** 1 cup natural cassava flour, cinnamon ½ teaspoon, 1 banana, 2 eggs, vanilla extract 1 teaspoon, baking powder 2 teaspoon, 2 tablespoons unrefined coconut oil, 1 ½ cup almond or coconut milk.

**Cooking instruction:** Preheat the waffle iron
Add all the ingredients and blend for about 30 seconds to 1 minute.
Pour onto the waffle iron the batter and cooked through. Remove when it becomes crispy and golden brown and Top with desired ingredients.

## 69. Pumpkin spiced chocolate slab

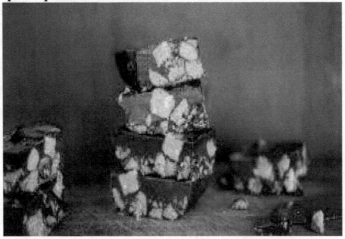

**Cooking time:**

**Ingredients:** 4 pumpkins spiced collagen bars, cut into squares.
vanilla powder 1 teaspoon
cocoa powder 1 cup
cocoa butter 1 cup
A salt
Sweetener

**Cooking instructions:** Add cocoa powder, butter in a saucepan and heat until completely melted. Now add chocolate powder, vanilla, salt and sweetener to taste.
Mix the ingredients, pour liquid chocolate in container and sprinkle the chopped pumpkin bar.
Place it into the fridge to set. When it's ready, slice chocolate slab into pieces and enjoy.

**Nutrition:**

Calories: 234

Carbohydrate: 9.4 gm

Fat: 20gm

Protein: 8gm

Fibre: 4 gm

## 70. Strawberry almond energy balls

This quick almond energy ball gives you a kick of energy easy to make a low carb diet.

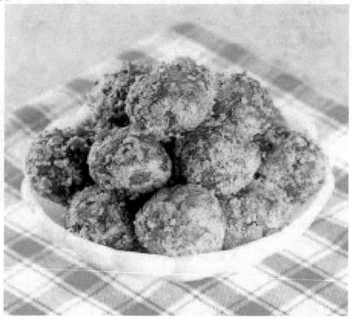

**Cooking time:** 1 hour

**Ingredients:** 1 cup pitted dates, 4 medium, strawberries sliced, ¾ cup almond, ½ cup oats, ½ cup coconut flakes.

**Instructions:** Combine all the above listed ingredients except coconut flakes, put them in food processor, and processed them until ground till it received thick consistency
Make small bowls from the thick paste and place them in the fridge to set for one hour

**Nutrition:**

calories 91

Fat: 8gm

Protein: 10%

Carbohydrate: 10gm

## 71. Brussels chips

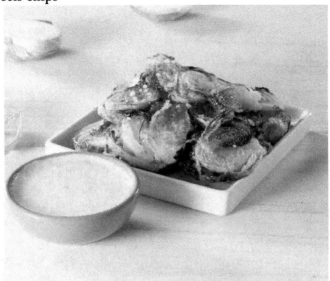

**Total cooking time:** 25 mins

**Ingredients:** 1 lb brussels sprouts thinly sliced, 2 tablespoon parmesan cheese, garlic powder 1 tablespoon, olive oil 1 tablespoon, salt, pepper, Caesar dressing.

**Cooking Instructions:** Preheat the oven at 400°F. Now in a bowl add brussels sprouts and toss them into the olive oil, parmesan, garlic powder, salt, pepper.
Spread these slices on baking tray and bake them for 10 minutes.
Serve them by adding Caesar dressing.

**Nutrition:**

Calories: 41,

Fat: 1g,

Fibre: 2g,

Carbohydrates: 1.5g,

Protein: 12mg,

Cholesterol: 0.0mg.

## 72. Avocado chips

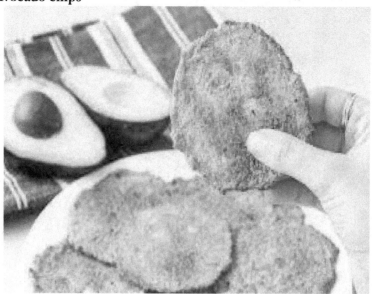

**Total cooking time:** 30 minutes

**Ingredients:** 1 large size avocado, ¾ cup grated parmesan, ½ teaspoon garlic powder, ½ teaspoon Italian seasonings, salt, black pepper, lime juice.

**Cooking procedure:**
Preheat the oven at 325°F. Place baking sheet in oven.
Now add mash avocado in bowl and stir it with remaining ingredients.
Now place a scoop of this mixture on a baking sheet and press them firmly.
Once it has done, bake the chips for about 20 minutes and let them cool.
Serve it and enjoy it as you want by adding more seasonings.

**Nutrition:**

Calories: 32,

Fat: 3g, Protein: 1g,

Cholesterol: 0.0mg,

Fibre:1g